Cancer Therapies
Awesome New Advances

by

Anna Rovid Spickler, DVM, Ph.D.

Biotech Publishing
A Division of
Plant Something Different, Inc.
Angleton, TX. USA

Cancer Therapies

Awesome New Advances

by Anna Rovid Spickler, DVM, Ph.D.

Published by Biotech Publishing
P. O. Box 1032
Angleton, TX. 77516-1032
(281) 369-2044

Copyright ©1998 by Biotech Publishing

Printing 10 9 8 7 6 5 4 3 2 1

Library of Congress Catalog Number   98-87754
Softcover   ISBN 1-880319-22-5

Publisher's Cataloging in Publication Data
Spickler, Anna Rovid
Cancer Therapies-Awesome New Advances
Includes glossary, bibliographical references, index
1. Cancer 2. Research 3. Treatment 4. Prevention
                     1998
RC 267

Cover, layout, and illustration
by Tammy Kay Crask

Contents

Section I. What is cancer?

Chapter 1: What is cancer? 1

Chapter 2: A brief review of genetics 9

Chapter 3: How mutations turn a normal cell
into a cancer cell 17

Chapter 4: Oncogenes - the cancer genes 25

Chapter 5: Tumor suppressor genes, the good guys 35

Section II. The treatment of cancer

Chapter 6: Traditional Therapies - surgery,
radiation, and chemotherapy 45

Chapter 7: Radiotherapy 49

Chapter 8: Chemotherapy -
The search for new drugs 61

Chapter 9: Tried and true anti-cancer drugs -
and some of their newer relatives 71

Chapter 10: The problems with drugs - side effects
and drug resistance 85

Chapter 11: Magic Bullets - targeting tumor cells
With antibodies and other carriers 97

Chapter 12: Circadian rhythms - how our internal
clocks affect cancer drugs 105

Chapter 13: Giving life-threatening doses of drugs -
high dose chemotherapy 109

Chapter 14: Manipulating growth factors 117

Chapter 15: Hormones and anti-hormones in
          cancer treatment   125

Chapter 16: Vitamins in cancer treatment   135

Chapter 17: Stopping cancer cells from spreading -
          prevention of metastasis   139

Chapter 18: Cutting off the supply lines- attacking
          normal cells to destroy the tumor   147

Chapter 19: Phototherapy - using light to destroy
          cancer   157

Chapter 20: Hyperthermia - turning up the heat   167

Chapter 21: Apoptosis - asking cancer cells
          to kill themselves   171

Chapter 22: The immune system   181

Chapter 23: How the immune system kills cancer
          cells - and how the cancer fights back   193

Chapter 24: Boosting the immune system to fight
          cancer   199

Chapter 25: Using immune cells and antibodies
          to treat tumors   207

Chapter 26: Cancer vaccines   217

Chapter 27: Gene therapy - a glimpse into the future   227

Chapter 28: Learning to prevent cancer   241

Epilogue   250
References   252
Glossary   278
Trade Names   283
Index   284

To Don...

Without you this book would never have been written.

Acknowledgments

The author would like to extend her grateful thanks to the many people at Biotech Publishing who have patiently read, critiqued, and otherwise helped with this book. Particular thanks go to Paige Pavlik, who spent many hours in the library finding scientific papers and suggested other useful ones, and to Carl Tant, who made this book possible. A special thanks also to my husband, Donald Spickler, who not only gave up his computer, but also spent endless hours reading the text as a non-biologist. The photo of liver metastasis on page 48 was supplied by Donna Tant, RN and James Maguine, M.D.

A Note from the Publisher

Is it possible for a person without training in biology to understand the complexities of cancer? Following the shocks of cancer diagnosis, the victim, family, and friends are plunged into confusing and often frightening world of big medicine. All too often medical specialists fail to explain fully the processes of treatments or alternatives possible.

Cruelly, in its own scientific ignorance, the popular news media often raises false hopes by reporting the results of early basic research as a promising new cancer treatment. The truth, as Dr. Spickler stresses here, is that most of the preliminary hopes do not pan out in later testing. Garbage on the internet adds to the dilemma of many victims.

We recognize that this book is somewhat longer and seems more technical than other titles in the ASB Series. It really isn't, but cancer treatment is a special world with its own language. The big words used to describe processes and treatment are unavoidable - they all have special meaning which the author has carefully explained as they are introduced. Follow her explanations with Tammy Crask's illustrations and you will soon gain understanding of the way things really are. The extensive glossary included will help further.

There are no miracle pills for instant cure. Even so, many new and experimental treatments offer hope for extended quality life. Hard choices ultimately often must be made by the patient and family. We hope the knowledge reviewed here will help make those choices on an intelligent informed basis.

THE AWESOME SCIENCE OF BIOLOGY SERIES

Welcome to the fourth volume of the Awesome Science of Biology Series!

Today, the science of biology is changing at a rate undreamed of only one or two decades ago. The theoretical laboratory research of a year ago suddenly becomes practical application. The new knowledge creates new subdivisions of biological science. It has become difficult for scientists, even biologists, to keep up with the changes. The task of understanding the new knowledge is almost insurmountable for the non-scientist. Yet, there is a pressing necessity to understand.

The new processes and technologies are described in scientific research literature which, even if accessible, is unfamiliar to the non-scientist. The technical terminology utilized in reporting research results is more often than not the equivalent of being addressed in a foreign language for the average layperson. The alternative is often only to obtain information from the popular press. Unfortunately, much of the information is presented by writers who, themselves, do not have a science background to understand the full implications of the processes, or are seeking dramatic subjects to capture the reader's attention and sell more copies of the publication.

The goal of the ASB SERIES is to explore the new knowledge with a scientifically qualified author who can translate the technical jargon of the research literature into terms understandable by those not specialized in the discipline. Our only sources of information are interviews with scientists themselves and peer-reviewed scientific literature. No information is based on the sensational stories often found in the popular press. The sources of information are properly cited in the text and a reference list with full details of publication is provided for those who might have interest in and access to it.

Long technical terms are often a turn-off for people who would otherwise like to further their scientific knowledge. We do not oversimplify and attempt to eliminate such terms because we live in a technical world and new words are continually coined to describe new processes. We do attempt to explain these terms in a manner the average reader can understand.

The ASB SERIES does not pretend to be an exhaustive survey of all the scientific literature about a particular topic. That is the proper domain of literature reviews published in scientific research journals or even in review books. We have, however, made every effort to review the most pertinent and, what we feel to be, the most important reports on a subject. Sometimes, these may not be the most recent. If, for example, a scientist made a major discovery and reported it in 1987, that work will be cited. While confirmation is recognized as being important, later "me too" reports by other scientists may not be mentioned. Where research results or interpretations differ and there is legitimate scientific disagreement, the ASB SERIES attempts to explain all viewpoints.

x

Chapter 1

What Is Cancer?

Cancer starts very small - in a single cell, in a few genes of that cell. However, those changes affect the cell profoundly, leading to more and more changes until, finally, the cancer cell looks and acts nothing like the cell from which it originated. In the next few chapters, we will examine the changes that occur in a normal cell to turn it into a cancer cell. Let's begin, however, with an overview of cancer: what cancer is, how cancers are named, how cancers develop, and why cancer is so deadly.

A cancer cell is simply a cell which has become capable of unlimited growth. The body makes new cells by splitting existing cells, making two cells out of one. Ordinarily, this process, called cell division, is under very strict control. But cancer cells have developed mutations in their genes which allow them to escape that control; they can divide constantly. Almost any cell in the body can turn into a cancer cell (with the exception of some cells which are incapable of dividing, such as mature nerve cells). Depending on the origins of the cell, and how the genes have been altered, cancers differ from each other. They differ in their speed of growth, their destructiveness, and their susceptibility to treatment. Certain cancers such as some kidney cancers and lung cancer are typically more aggressive; others are usually slower to grow. Even the same type of cancer varies from patient to patient, and from month to month (untreated tumors typically grow more aggressive as time goes on).

What's in a name?

Cancers are usually named for where they originate (although they may occasionally be named after a physician or scientist - such as Hodgkins lymphoma or Kaposi's sarcoma - or by their appearance, such as hairy cell leukemia). For example, glioblastomas develop from glial cells (support cells for nerves) and melanomas have their origins in melanocytes, pigment producing cells found in the skin. A complete name for a cancer often includes the terms carcinoma or sarcoma.

Carcinomas are cancers that develop from epithelial tissues, layers of cells which typically cover body and organ surfaces and form glands. Carcinomas are the most common types of adult cancers; they include such cancers as breast cancer and colon cancer. Sarcomas develop from what are called mesenchymal tissues; these include muscle, bone and other tissues. Leukemia is a general term for various cancers of the red and white blood cells; this term is used when these cancer cells are found as individual cells in the blood. When white blood cell cancers grow as solid clumps of cells, they are called lymphomas.

A tumor is a lump or "growth," a mass of abnormal cells. Not all tumors are cancers. A lump could be a benign tumor which is not cancer, but simply a clump of misplaced cells, or a malignant tumor, which is cancer. What is the difference between them? Basically, it is in the speed of their growth and their tendency to spread to their surroundings.

In a benign tumor, the cells divide relatively slowly. Benign tumors may grow, but they grow slowly and do not spread into normal tissues. In fact, they are often contained within a capsule, a surrounding shell produced by neighboring normal cells. Their cells usually bear some resemblance to their cell of origin. Benign tumors are rarely fatal unless they have been ignored to the point where they compress the surrounding tissues and interfere with the normal functioning of the body. For example, benign tumors form many of the skin lumps and bumps we get as we grow older or the fatty lumps called lipomas on your dog.

Malignant tumors (cancers) tend to grow quickly and aggressively. They invade their surroundings, crawling between the normal cells surrounding them and sometimes even traveling to distant sites in the body. They are not stopped when they meet boundaries that normal cells would respect. One boundary, for example, is a skin barrier called the basement membrane (Figure 1.1). The basement membrane is a thin layer of proteins which separates an outer layer of epithelial (covering) cells from an inner layer of cells and proteins called connective tissue. A normal epithelial skin cell will divide when new skin cells are needed, but its progeny would never cross the basement membrane. A benign epithelial cell tumor would also remain above the basement membrane. An epithelial cancer would, however, simply penetrate through the basement membrane, and continue to divide in the connective tissue below.

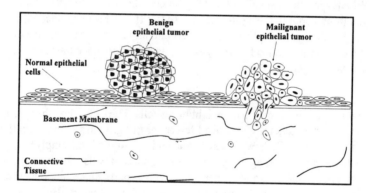

Figure 1.1. Malignant tumors penetrate through normal barriers such as the basement membrane.

What makes a cancer cell different from a normal cell?

A cell becomes a cancer cell through mutations, changes in its genes. Those changes alter the cell in two simple, but profound ways: it can divide without being told to divide and it becomes immortal.

A common misconception is that all cells in the body are immortal. Not so. Like people, normal cells have definite life spans. A cell's lifespan, however, seems to be measured by how many times it divides. A normal cell can reproduce itself only a limited number of times; after that, it dies (Levine, 1997; Ehrenstein, 1998). Cancer cells have mutations that allow them to escape this death (Ehrenstein, 1998). In a sense, they are the immortal Dracula of the cellular world. And, like vampires, they pay no attention to the normal rules of their society. Normal cell division is controlled by some very strict rules. In general, cells only divide when the body is growing (during development and childhood) or where cells have died and need to be replaced. Normal cells wait until they receive growth factors, proteins sent to a cell which "tell" it to divide. Even if a cell receives growth factors, however, other controls may prevent cell division. One important control is contact with neighboring cells. Whenever a normal cell is touching its neighbors, cell division stops. If you think about it, this system makes sense. If a cell is in contact with its neighbors, there are plenty of cells around and no new cells are needed. If a cell is surrounded by empty space, its neighbors have died and there is a need to replace them.

Cancer cells have, however, lost this control. They don't seem to notice that they are in contact with neighboring cells. Through other changes in the cell, they generally also need fewer (or no) growth factors from the rest of the body. So now, this immortal and uninhibited cell simply begins to divide and divide again, growing into a mass of cells. This difference between normal cells and cancer cells becomes particularly obvious when cells are taken out of the body and grown in the laboratory. Both cancer cells and normal cells can be grown for a time inside containers with a supply of nutrients. Normal cells divide until they form a layer of cells on the bottom of the container, then stop dividing. They do not grow over each other. If some of the cells are taken out, the remaining cells can once again divide until they form a layer of cells - but, again, they stop. Cancer cells, on the other hand, ignore their neighbors; they continue to divide, even when they are growing on top of other cells. Rather than a smooth sheet of cells, cancer cells often form a sheet with thick clumps and lumps. Inside the organism, this rapid, disorganized growth is also apparent. In normal tissues, there are neat bundles of cells, separated and organized and served by an orderly array of arteries, veins, and nerves. In cancerous tumors, the cells are loosely connected and haphazardly distributed, each cell competing with the next for its share of space and nutrients.

As a cancer cell's genes change to allow uncontrolled growth, the cells also change in appearance (Figure 1.2). As they become immortal, they also begin to look more primitive. They begin to resemble immature cells which specialize in making new cells, and not the mature cells of their origins. Cancer cells also look different from each other, even in a single tumor. As they divide, they accumulate mutations, so that one cell can have an entirely different set of mutations than its neighbors. This results in a set of cells that often varies wildly in size and shape.

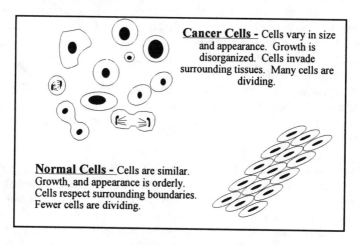

Figure 1.2. Characteristics of cancer cells and normal cells.

How cancers change, grow and spread

Cancers start as a single mutant cell, undetectable by touch or sight. This cell divides repeatedly and, eventually, the group of cells becomes large enough to detect as a lump. As the lump grows beyond a certain size, it develops its own blood supply. The cancer cells stimulate the blood vessels around them to start growing into the tumor, forming a new network of blood vessels inside the tumor itself. The cancer cells inside the tumor are dependent on these blood vessels for the oxygen and nutrients they need for life. These new blood vessels do not, however, grow as normal blood vessels do - their structure is much less organized (for example, capillaries may sprout from arteries of any size) and they tend to be kinked, with rather leaky walls which may break open and bleed (Hall, 1995; Cheville, 1993). These vessels are often too small for some blood cells to pass through them (Hall, 1995). Sometimes, blood flow shuts down or even reverses itself (Hall, 1995). Partly because these blood vessels are so odd, and partly because the cancer cells grow faster than the blood vessels, oxygen and nutrient delivery is not as efficient as it is to normal tissues. As a result, some cancer cells die. Clumps of dead cells become mixed among the living cells. Other cells continue to divide, but more slowly because their oxygen and nutrient needs are not being fully met. These pockets of slowly dividing tumor cells can become resistant to some cancer treatments.

As the cancer grows, its cells also develop the ability to crawl away from the main tumor. Some of these cells may reach blood vessels or lymphatic vessels (which carry a fluid called lymph back to the blood). Cells which enter the blood can be carried throughout the body to seed other tissues with tumor cells; this is called metastasis and is deadly (Figure 1.3). Fortunately, most metastatic cells die in the blood and never reach a suitable site to establish a new tumor colony. One estimate is that fewer than one in 10,000 cancer cells manages to leave the blood and form a new tumor (Rischer, 1995). Given enough time and enough cells, however, some will make it. Metastasis is the reason that early detection of cancer is so important. Once they have dispersed throughout the body, cancer cells are very difficult to eradicate. No longer is it a case of removing a single lump of abnormal cells; now, it is a matter of trying to destroy cells which are hiding in the lungs, the bone marrow, and the brain. Sometimes these cells are in groups so small that they escape detection until they, too send out invaders to new tissues.

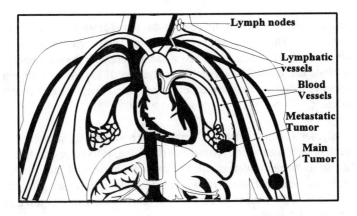

Figure 1.3. Metastatic tumor in the lung, developed from a tumor originally in the arm.

How cancer kills

And yet, finally, why is a mass of cells, even an undisciplined mass of cells, so dangerous? In other words, how does cancer kill? There is no simple answer to this question. Malignant tumors seem to destroy the body not in one way, but in many. The most obvious is when they destroy an organ by crushing the surrounding cells or interfering with the organ's functions. For example, picture a growing mass of cells within an enclosed space such as the brain: normal cells will simply be crushed by the increasing pressure. A cancer near the heart might interfere with the pumping and return of blood. Another might disrupt the kidney's orderly structure to the point where it can no longer filter blood and shuts down, trapping poisons in the body.

Cancer cells also starve the body by using all of the available nutrients for their own growth. In fact, cancer cells aggressively compete for more than their fair share of nutrients (Rischer, 1995; Cheville, 1993). This can drain the host of proteins until the muscles shrivel and finally even such vital organs as the liver and pancreas diminish (Cheville, 1993). To make it worse, cancers often result in loss of appetite, possibly through a direct effect on the brain (Cheville, 1993).

Cancers can also prevent the cells of the blood from carrying out their normal jobs. They can suppress the immune system and leave a person vulnerable to infections. They may also interfere with the components of the blood that control blood clotting (Cheville, 1993). As a result, either excessive blood clotting or bleeding is possible. Anemia is also common in cancer.

Finally, some tumors can make hormones or hormone-like substances that interfere with normal body functions (Cheville, 1993). For example, one dangerous hormone drains calcium from the bones and raises calcium levels in the blood. Excessive calcium in the blood can cause a variety of symptoms, from nausea to coma. The damage increases as the cancer spreads to more sites.

Chapter 2

A Brief Review of Genetics

In modern cancer treatment and diagnosis, knowledge of cancer genes is becoming ever more important. Genetic abnormalities can predict the success of a treatment, allow patients to be included or excluded from trials of new treatments, and even form a basis for new gene therapies. To understand cancer thoroughly, you need to have a basic understanding of genes. This section is, therefore, for those who might need a short refresher course on DNA.

The basics of genetics

We don't often think very deeply about how our body runs itself. It just seems to work- somehow. But, as we look more deeply into the body, we discover layer upon layer of complexity. The human body is made of organs such as the kidneys or heart, each specialized to do a particular job. Organs are built out of tissues, groups of specialized cells (such as muscle tissue or bone). Within the tissues are the cells, the basic building blocks of the body. Ultimately, the cells are in charge. Each cell has a particular job to do. Individual cells communicate with each other and, together, they keep the body functioning. Each cell contains genes which provide all the information needed to run that cell. So if you really think about it, it is our genes that are responsible for keeping the body running smoothly.

Genes are simply pieces of DNA which carry the information to make proteins. They are found in the nucleus of a cell, packaged into the chromosomes. Human cells have 46 chromosomes, including two "sex chromosomes," the X and Y chromosomes which determine whether an individual is male or female. The rest of the chromosomes come in pairs; each cell contains 2 copies of each chromosome, one inherited from each parent. Each pair of chromosomes has the same genes; however, the two copies of each gene are not necessarily identical. Some genes, such as those which determine eye color, come in a variety of forms. Other genes, however, are essential to the body in one particular form. These genes are either identical or extremely similar between healthy individuals. For example, the genes that make hemoglobin, the molecule which carries oxygen in the blood, cannot change much without causing disease; all hemoglobin genes in healthy people look the same. One advantage to carrying two copies of such genes is that if one is damaged somehow, the cell can often continue to function normally, using the other. Most of the cancer genes that we will be concerned with fall into this category.

Although all cells carry the same chromosomes and the same genetic information, different cells use different bits of that information. For instance, only the cells which go on to become red blood cells use the hemoglobin gene and only the cells which form the iris of the eye use the genes which control eye pigment. In any given cell, at any given time, some genes are active, or "on" and others are inactive.

The structure of genes -
and how mutations change that structure

A gene is a rather amazingly simple thing. Every gene contains nothing more than four different chemicals called bases, put together in a specific order on a structure which supports them and glues them together (Figure 2.1). These bases are called adenine, guanine, cytosine, and thymine. For convenience, they are usually abbreviated as A, G, C and T. A gene is simply a specific, unique sequence of bases. You could make any gene just by knowing the order of its bases. To make human insulin, for example, you would string together ATGGCCCTGTGGA .... until you reached the end of the gene. To make estrogen, you would string together a different sequence. For the skin protein keratin, yet another sequence. And so on.

These bases are strung in a row onto a support structure, a "backbone" or scaffolding of sugar and phosphate groups. Actually, the DNA molecule contains two parallel strings of bases. The bases face each other inward, and each interacts with the base across from it. In this structure, there are some limits on which bases can interact with each other. Adenine (A) can only pair with thymine (T) and guanine (G) can only pair with cytosine

(C). So one string (known as the coding strand) contains the genetic information for insulin; the other is gibberish whose base sequence is dictated by the coding strand. When the gene is read by the cellular machinery, the two strands briefly separate, and the coding strand is read; the strands are then allowed to interact again.

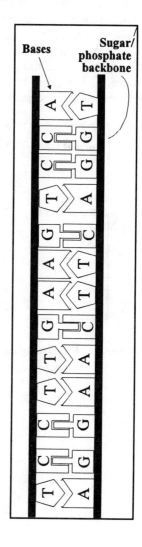

Figure 2.1. The structure of DNA.

When the sequence of bases in a gene is altered, it is called a mutation (Figure 2.2). A base might be left out, or an extra one put in or one base changed to another kind (for example, an adenine replaced by a cytosine). In some cases, a mutation may make only a minor change (or no change) in the meaning of the gene; in others cases, it may completely destroy its usefulness. Some of the most dramatic mutations are breaks in the chromosomes. In some cases, the broken chromosome is re-attached, but to the wrong chromosome! Such changes can join two different genes together, creating a composite gene which does something completely unexpected. It can also destroy genes, or make them either more or less active. Chromosome breaks where one chromosome is reattached to another are fairly common in some leukemias (Look, 1997).

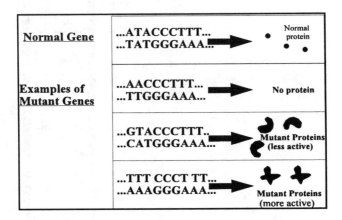

Figure 2.2. Examples of mutations in a gene.

How genes are turned into proteins

It is important to understand that genes are vital only as sources of information. They cannot leave the chromosome or physically perform any of the duties of a cell. Genes control the cell's functions by controlling the production of proteins. Each gene carries the information to make a particular protein. When a certain set of genes is active, those proteins are made, and the cell acts in one particular way. When a different set of genes is active, a different set of proteins is made and the cell acts differently. The proteins perform all of the functions needed in a cell. Proteins manufacture substances needed by the body, control what goes into and comes out of a cell, communicate with other cells - and even regulate other genes!

A gene is turned into a protein by translating one language, the language of the gene, into another language, the language of proteins. For this reason, the process is called "translation." In a gene, the sequence of bases has a meaning. A protein, however, is made up of molecules called amino acids, not bases. There are 20 different amino acids, and the order in which they are strung together determines what protein it is. So to turn a gene's information into protein, the cell must take a sequence of bases and turn it into the corresponding sequence of amino acids. There are rules which make the translation simple. The most important rule is that every sequence of 3 bases corresponds to an amino acid. It's something like the secret codes of spy novels. Know the base sequence and the code, and you can translate it into the amino acids.

The cell has an elaborate, elegant set of machinery to do this translation (Figure 2.3). In an animal cell, the genes are contained inside the nucleus and separated from the cytoplasm by a membrane barrier. The protein synthesis machinery is, however, located inside the cytoplasm. To carry information from the nucleus to the cytoplasm, a copy is made of a gene; this copy is called messenger RNA. (It's like wanting to use a recipe from a library book that you can't check out. You copy the recipe on a copy machine, then take the copy with you and leave the original in the library.) Messenger RNA, incidentally, is a little different from DNA. It has only one strand, not two, and the bases are slightly different: a base called uracil is substituted for thymine.

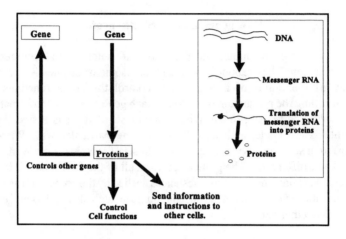

Figure 2.3. Proteins are made from genes, and control all of the activities of a cell.

Messenger RNA is only made from genes which are active. Which genes are active, and how active they are, is controlled by a group of proteins known as transcription factors. The transcription factors actually control how many copies of messenger RNA are made from any given gene. The more messenger RNA, the more protein will be made from that gene (Figure 2.4). Each messenger RNA molecule leaves the nucleus and goes to the cytoplasm. In the cytoplasm, an elaborate set of machinery translates the messenger RNA into the corresponding protein. Each copy of messenger RNA can be translated over and over (though they eventually wear out), making several copies of each protein. These proteins then carry out all of the functions of the cell. As we will see later, some cancer treatments attempt to shut off abnormal genes by interfering with the messenger RNA or other steps during protein production.

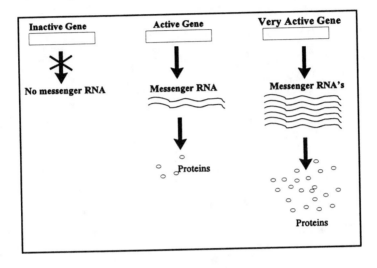

Figure 2.4.

How a cell passes down its genes -
DNA duplication and cell division

Whenever the animal body needs new cells, it stimulates a cell to split into two cells. To function properly, each new cell must inherit a full set of all of the chromosomes, in duplicate like its parent. The original cell (the "parent" cell) does this by making an extra copy of its chromosomes, then making sure that each new cell (known as the "daughter" cells or "progeny") has one copy of every chromosome. Since the DNA molecule is double stranded, copying chromosomes to pass down to daughter cells is quite easy. Remember that the chromosome has an adenine across from every thymine, a cytosine across from every guanine. So by knowing the sequence of bases on one strand, you would automatically know the sequence on the other. When a cell is going to divide, it simply splits each chromosome in half, and regenerates the other half of the DNA strand, using the rules of base pairing. Then one copy of each chromosome moves to each half of the cell (guided by a structure called the mitotic spindle), and it splits in two. End result: two daughter cells with exactly the same genes.

Chapter 3

How mutations turn a normal cell into a cancer cell

Until fairly recently, the causes of cancer were very much a mystery. Slowly, we are learning more. In the first chapter, we discussed how a cancer cell begins to grow out of control, eventually forming a malignant tumor and possibly metastasizing throughout the body. How does a cell go wrong? What changes start this deadly process? Hopes for cancer prevention, and even for cures, may lie in the knowledge of those origins.

It takes time for a normal cell to develop into a cancer cell. It doesn't happen in one step or in a single mutation. Instead, normal cells seem to progress to cancer cells in a two-stage process (Figure 3.1): those two stages are called initiation and promotion (Cheville, 1993). During initiation, a cell is freed from the normal controls that would suppress its division. Promotion stimulates the altered cell to actually divide. Initiation usually occurs by a change to a gene; these mutated "cancer genes" are called oncogenes. Promotion may be caused by mutations in the cell's genes, but it can also occur when a change in the cell's environment encourages it to grow. Anything which stimulates cell growth, such as excessive amounts of growth factors or nutrients, could act as a cancer promoter.

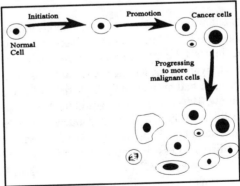

Figure 3.1. A cancer cell is made in a two-stage process, then continues to accumulate mutations.

Once they have mutated, cancer cells continue to accumulate mutations. Some researchers estimate that any cancer cell plucked from a tumor would have at least half a dozen changes in its genes (Hartwell, 1997). The cells make extra copies of certain genes, often lose or gain whole chromosomes, and are prone to further mutations in their genes (Hartwell, 1997). Some cancer cells die from these mutations. Other changes, however, allow the cells to adapt to new environments. For example, cancer cells can mutate and become resistant to drugs designed to kill them. Mutations also allow cancer cells to become more aggressive as time goes on; the most competitive cells leave more descendants.

What causes cancer mutations

Some mutated genes are inherited at birth, but most mutations occur during the life of an individual. Only five percent of cancers seem to be caused by inherited mutations (Perera, 1997). The other 95 percent are caused by new mutations, combined with a susceptibility to cancer (Perera, 1997). Susceptibility to cancer can be affected by many factors from diet and lifestyle to the specific genetic makeup of an individual. Likewise, many environmental factors can cause mutations. Some of the more important are radiation, chemical carcinogens, and certain viruses.

Radiation

Radiation is one well-known source of mutations and increased cancer risk (Perera, 1997). While massive doses of radiation can kill immediately, lower doses can alter the structure of our DNA and cause cancer. The survivors of the atomic bombs at Hiroshima and Nagaskai, for example, have had an unusually high risk for leukemia and other cancers (Berkow, 1992). There is a natural tendency, when we think of radiation, to think of atomic blasts and nuclear disasters such as the meltdown at Chernobyl. Fortunately, few of us are exposed to such sources of radiation. Less dramatic types of radiation are, however, common in our everyday lives. Ultraviolet radiation from the sun damages the DNA of our skin cells. This is why we get a tan: skin cells are frantically making a sunshade of pigments to protect their DNA from further damage by the sun. A radioactive gas, radon, is found in mines and some homes. Excessive exposure to X-rays can cause mutations. Even if we avoid all artificial sources of radiation, our cells are constantly bombarded with natural cosmic radiation from the universe surrounding us. It is sobering to realize that short of locking ourselves in a small radiation- proof room, there is no way to completely avoid exposure to radiation. We can minimize the damage by reducing our x-ray exposure to only that which is medically necessary, being very careful with radioactive materials, and using sun screens, but we cannot reduce our exposure to zero.

Some scientists, however, question whether we need to fear radiation quite as much as we do. Although researchers know that, with larger doses of radiation, increased radiation leads to an increased risk of cancer, no one yet knows how the body reacts to exposure to very small doses. Some scientists say that any exposure is harmful; others, that our bodies can cope with very small amounts. In the meantime, government regulatory agencies have set maximum exposure levels for the general public and different levels for people who work with radiation.

Chemical carcinogens

Chemicals can also cause changes in DNA that increase the risk of cancer. These chemicals are called carcinogens. The first known carcinogen was discovered by Sir Percival Potts, who noticed that English chimney sweeps had an unusually high risk of getting cancer of the scrotum (Cheville, 1993). Eventually, the carcinogen in soot was identified as the chemical dibenzanthracene. Similar chemicals are also found in cigarette smoke (Cheville, 1993). Cigarette smoke is, in fact, a notorious source of carcinogens; at least 43 are known (Perera, 1997; Rischer, 1995). Tobacco use has been linked to lung cancers, as well as cancers of the esophagus, bladder, and head and neck (Berkow, 1992). There are many other carcinogens in the world. Many different substances in our diet, drugs, and pollutants may be carcinogens (Perera, 1997). In fact, chemicals which can mutate our DNA may be surprisingly common. As many as half of all chemicals, either natural or man-made (Ames 1990) may be capable of damaging our DNA!

Some of us may be more susceptible to chemicals and radiation than others

According to recent research, some of us seem to be much more susceptible to carcinogens and radiation than others. F.P. Perera (1997) recently described the relative risks for various groups of people. Infants and children, for example, seem to be particularly at risk. Their bodies tend to absorb and retain environmental toxins more than adults. Because they are growing, their cells are also dividing more often than adults; rapid cell division gives each cell less time to correct mutations. Adolescence and early adulthood also seems to be a dangerous time. For example, women who were in their teens during the atomic bomb blasts had the highest risk of breast cancer from the radiation. The risk of lung cancer for women who began smoking under the age of 25 is almost four times as high as the risk for women who started smoking over 25. Some think that the elderly, who have decreased immune function and lower DNA repair rates, may also be more susceptible to carcinogens. There even seems to be a sex difference: women who smoke are 1.7 to 3 times as likely to develop lung cancer as men who smoke the same amount. Finally, there is individual variability. For example, when a group of people was exposed to the same amount of chemicals in fossil fuel, they had different amounts of damage to their DNA (Perera, 1997). All of these differences in reaction seem to be greatest at low levels of exposure to carcinogens. At high levels, everyone's risk becomes great.

Cancer viruses

Viruses can also cause cancer. Only a few types of viruses, however, seem to be the culprits - and only in specific types of cancers. Of the approximately 20 groups of viruses, only some members of five groups (the retroviruses, herpes viruses, papillomaviruses, hepadnaviruses, and polyomaviruses) have been associated with cancers. Some viruses which have been linked to human cancers are papillomaviruses in cervical cancer, a herpes virus with Kaposi's sarcoma, a retrovirus with leukemia, and hepatitis B virus with liver cancer (Rickinson, 1995; Kledal, 1997). The Epstein-Barr virus (the cause of mononucleosis) is also associated with various cancers in some parts of the world (Rickinson, 1995). How most of these viruses cause cancer is still pretty much a mystery. One fascinating group of cancer viruses has, however, revealed some of its secrets.

These viruses, known as the oncogenic retroviruses, are distant relatives of the AIDS virus. They can cause feline leukemia in cats, one form of lymphoma in cattle, a leukemia in humans, and a variety of tumors in chickens (Fenner, 1987). When they infect a cell, the oncogenic retroviruses insert a copy of their genes into the cell's own chromosomes. These genes can cause cancer in two very different ways (Fenner).

Retroviruses of one type carry oncogenes. By delivering an oncogene to a normal cell, they can turn the cell into a cancer cell almost immediately (Figure 3.2). Infection with these viruses is possibly the quickest way of getting cancer; in some animals, tumors can develop in two weeks after infection (Fenner, 1987). Fortunately, these viruses do not seem to infect humans, although some affect other animals such as cats and chickens. Another type of oncogenic retrovirus wreaks havoc by damaging the genes of infected cells (Figure 3.3). For example, once in a while, the retrovirus may insert itself into the middle of an active gene and destroy it. In other situations, it could make the cell's genes more active. This group of oncogenic retroviruses does not, however, carry oncogenes. Unlike their nastier relatives, they cause cancer in only a few of those infected by the virus, and only after a long period of infection. In essence, some who are infected with the virus simply get unlucky.

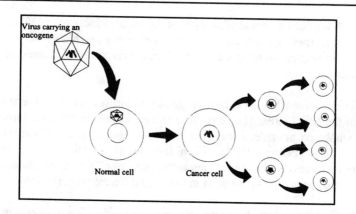

Figure 3.2. Some oncogenic retroviruses carry oncogenes which turn normal cells into cancer cells.

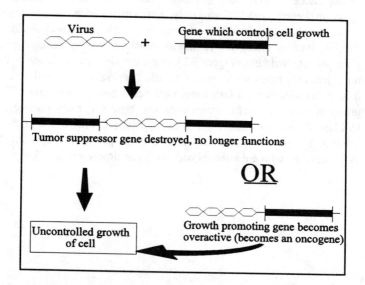

Figure 3.3. Some oncogenic retroviruses can accidentally land near important genes and alter them, initiating cancer.

The cancers associated with viruses are, however, preventable if infection with the virus can be prevented. In fact, one notable success in cancer prevention has been with a very contagious chicken herpes virus called the Marek's disease virus. This virus causes lymphomas and sarcomas in chickens. Vaccination against the Marek's disease virus can prevent this type of lymphoma in chickens (Fenner, 1987).

Hope for our genes - how mutations can be fixed before they cause trouble

After reading the preceding sections, the picture for our genes might look quite gloomy. We are surrounded by radiation, by chemical carcinogens, by cancer viruses, all fully capable of damaging our DNA. In fact, Dr. Bruce Ames (1990) estimates that the genes of human cells are damaged approximately 10,000 times every day. Why don't all of those damaged cells go on to become cancer cells? And how does anyone escape getting cancer, if this is true? The answer lies in the fact that I have, so far, only presented you with half of the story. The truth is that normal cells have a way to fight back - they have repair mechanisms for DNA damage.

There are many enzymes whose jobs are to repair damaged DNA in a cell. Some enzymes remove damaged pieces of DNA and fill in the gap with the proper bases, using the opposite strand of DNA as a guide. Other repair enzymes scan the chromosomes for mismatched bases (for example, an adenine paired with a cytosine). When a mismatch is discovered, the enzymes remove the wrong base, and replace it with the correct one. Damage to the repair systems themselves can be a real problem. People with a disease called xeroderma pigmentosum have defects in DNA repair and are unusually susceptible to genetic damage from UV light and to skin cancers (Lewin, 1990; Cheville, 1993).

Now, the bad news. Unfortunately, the repair enzymes do not seem to be able to keep up with the amount of DNA damage being done every day (Ames, 1990). Picture even an extremely efficient repair enzyme that allows only a single mutation to slip by each day. In two days, there will be two mutations in the body; in a week, seven, and in a year, 365. Fortunately, many of these mutations will be harmless ones which don't change the amino acid sequence, or "meaning" of the chromosomal messages. Some will occur in cells which are at the end of their life cycle and about to die anyway (for example, in a skin cell about to be sloughed off). Some will be in inactive genes, or in regions of the chromosome which do not contain genes. Other mutations will be changes to genes that cause the cell to die. But a few may be mutations in oncogenes. It is these mutations that have the potential to initiate the deadly changes that wait for a cancer promoter.

There are other reasons that all cells don't go on to become cancer cells. One of the most important is that genes known as tumor suppressor genes stop division in cells with mutations. We will look at specific tumor suppressor genes and oncogenes in the next two chapters.

Chapter 4

Oncogenes - the cancer genes

Until recently, the genes involved in cancer seemed very mysterious. Biologists knew that some cancer-causing viruses carried oncogenes. They also knew that the same genes were sometimes mutated in tumors which were not associated with viruses, but no one seemed to know what the oncogenes actually did. Recently, however, scientists have begun to solve the mystery. They have discovered that many cancer genes develop from the genes which control cell division. Some of these mutated genes, oncogenes, stimulate the development of cancer. Others, called tumor suppressor genes, prevent cancers until they are destroyed by mutations. To understand these genes, and how they interact, you will need to know a little about how cells send messages from one part of the cell to another.

Internal communications in cells - how different parts of the cell talk to each other

A cell might look quiet on the outside, but inside, at the molecular level, it is a hive of activity. Every moment, small factories (the mitochondria) are generating energy. Genes are being copied into messenger RNA. Proteins, fats and carbohydrates are being manufactured and transported. Others are being broken down. Messages are being sent to other cells, and received from other cells. All of this activity is highly coordinated: it is controlled by internal messages, signals being sent constantly from one part of the cell to another. Often, messages come from outside the cell as well, received and transmitted internally by molecules called receptors which are located on the cell surface (Figure 4.1).

The internal messages of cells ("signals") are complex, and as yet we understand only a little about them. In general, what happens is that first one molecule (perhaps a receptor on a cell surface, or one inside the cell which monitors internal conditions) is changed. This molecule then changes another molecule, which then changes another, and so on, until the last molecule actually carries out some task (Figure 4.1). Often (but not always) this change alters the activity of genes. The molecules involved in these pathways are often enzymes, special proteins which can make other molecules react with each other or split molecules apart. Other types of molecules are also used as messengers. A common signal is a change in the concentration of calcium in the cell: cells can hold calcium atoms inside special compartments, then release them to the cytoplasm, or suddenly allow calcium from outside the cell to enter. In a nutshell, there are a wide variety of signals, all sent by molecules, and all saying something meaningful to a part of the cell.

It would be misleading, however, to give the impression that each signal is sent in a straight line to the target within the cell. Signals branch to send messages to two or more targets and converge from different sources. In the end, if all of the signaling pathways within a cell were to be mapped out, the pattern would probably look like a web built by a mad spider, lines converging and splitting and interweaving. How the cell itself sorts out all of these messages and keeps them straight will undoubtedly be a mystery for some time.

Some of the most important signals in a cell are those that control when it divides. Many of the molecules involved in these signals have turned out to be oncogenes.

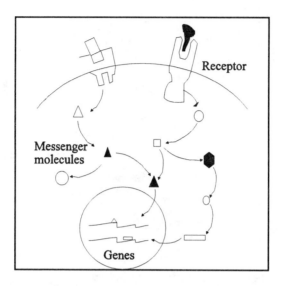

Figure 4.1. Signals sent from cell receptors, by messenger molecules.

The cell cycle and the control of normal cell division

Probably the most important events in the development of cancer are mutations in genes that control cell division. Many of these genes control a cell's progress through something called the cell cycle (Figure 4.2). The cell cycle is like a map of a cell's life stages. At any given time, a cell will be in one of the four stages of the cell cycle. In the stage known as G1, the cell is actively performing its normal functions, but it is not making new cells. Most cells in the body are in this stage, most of the time. When they are stimulated to grow, some cells enter the other three stages of the cycle, which are concerned with cell division. First, they move from G1 to a stage known as S, for DNA Synthesis. In this stage, the cell copies its DNA in preparation for cell division. After S, the cell enters a third stage, G2, in which it prepares further for cell division. Finally, in stage M, which is very brief, it actually divides. (Cell division of this sort is known as mitosis, which is where the M comes from). After cell division, the cell returns to G1, and either rests, or goes through the cycle and divides again. The cell cycle is often, but not always, shorter in tumor cells (Cheville, 1993).

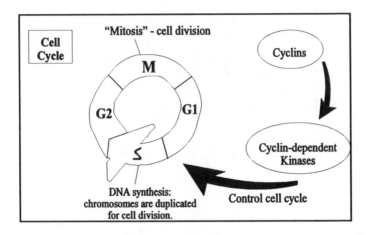

Figure 4.2. The cell cycle is controlled by cyclins.

A cell's progress through the cell cycle is controlled by a group of proteins known as the cyclins. There are several different cyclins; the amount of each cyclin increases and decreases in a regular pattern, as a cell moves from one stage to the next. For example, cyclin D1 increases as a cell prepares to enter the S stage of the cycle. Only when the right cyclins are at the right level in a cell will it enter the next stage. These guardian proteins control other proteins in the cell, known as cyclin-dependent kinases, which actually do the work of driving the cell through the cell cycle. In a sense, the cyclins act like symphony conductors, guiding the orchestra through a very complicated piece of music, in this case, the cell cycle.

In some cancer cells, it appears that some of the cell cycle genes, both the cyclins and the cyclin-dependent kinases, have been mutated. These changes stimulate the cell to perpetually divide. One particularly important cyclin in cancer is cyclin D1 (Marx, 1994). It is active at a critical time in the cell's cycle, when the decision is made to commit to cell division and enter the S phase. Cyclin D1 is mutated in some cancers. Another potential oncogene is cyclin E, which is also active during the G1 stage. The amount of cyclin E protein is higher than normal in some breast cancer cells (Marx, 1994). In fact, the concentration of cyclin E in a cell increases as breast cancers become more aggressive. Cyclin E may also be involved in lung, colon, and ovarian cancers. One of the cyclin dependent kinases, known as Cdk4, is also increased in some cancers (Marx, 1994). Other cyclins, and cyclin-dependent kinases, may also be involved in cancer development. Some genetic treatments for cancer attempt to turn off some of these oncogenes.

The checkpoints

At critical points in the cell cycle, between the four stages, there are regulatory systems known as checkpoints. The checkpoints stop the cyclins and interrupt the cell cycle when there has been DNA damage. They also interrupt the cycle when cells have not finished all of the tasks which will allow them to successfully complete the next stage of the cycle (Paulovich, 1997). Essentially, they stop cells from proceeding into the next stage unless everything in the cell is ready for the next stage. For example, a tumor suppressor, p53, stops the cycle in G1 when it senses DNA damage (Levine, 1997). Many other tumor suppressor proteins, discussed later, are also part of the checkpoints.

Why checkpoints fail

Often, however, cancer cells with DNA damage continue blindly through the cell cycle, oblivious to the checkpoints. Why don't checkpoints always stop damaged cells from dividing? The answer seems to be complicated. First, sometimes they simply make mistakes, and allow a cell to continue when it should be stopped (Paulovich, 1997).A second reason is that, after a time, the checkpoints may allow a cell to resume progress through the cycle even though the damage remains unrepaired; the cell seems to have become accustomed to the damage and sees it as something normal (Paulovich, 1997). Perhaps the most common reason, however, is that the checkpoint mechanisms have been mutated themselves (Paulovich, 1997). We will discuss these mutations with the tumor suppressor genes.

Growth factors

In normal cells, the cyclins do not act on their own; they are controlled by growth factors, hormones and other growth-stimulating proteins. These proteins are usually manufactured by one type of cell and sent to a different type of cell. They attach to receptors on the cell and send signals inside which, ultimately, control the cyclins and stimulate cell division (Figure 4.3). Altered growth factors and growth factor receptors often show up either as oncogenes or as contributors to the growth of cancers. Many cancer cells, for example, carry too many copies of the epidermal growth factor (EGF) receptor on their surfaces (Zalutsky, 1997; Barinaga, 1997b). The *HER-2/neu* protein, a protein related to the EGF receptor, has also been found in excess in many cancers, particularly aggressive ones (Viloria Petit, 1997). Treatments which suppress signals from growth factors have been able to slow the growth of some cancers. These treatments will be discussed in chapter 14.

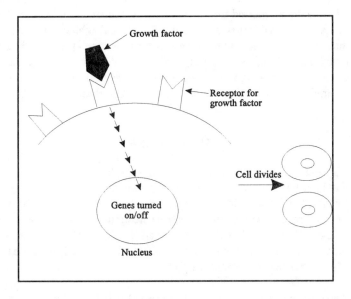

Figure 4.3. Growth factors stimulate cells to divide.

Internal signaling molecules as oncogenes

When growth factors or other cell stimulants send signals inside the cells, internal molecules must transmit those signals. Some of those internal signaling molecules, not surprisingly, have turned out to be oncogenes. One of the more commonly mutated oncogenes in tumors is called *Ras* (Barinaga, 1997b). The Ras protein is part of a signaling pathway which usually leads to cell growth (Barinaga, 1995). There are three different *Ras* genes; approximately 25 to 30 percent of tumors have a mutation in at least one of them (Barinaga 1997b). Mutations in signaling molecules similar to *Ras* can turn them into oncogenes, as well (Ehrenstein, 1998). Knowledge of *Ras* function has turned out to be helpful for cancer treatment. In some tumors, drugs which can suppress *Ras* can block the growth of the cancer (Barinaga, 1997b). Some drugs work by preventing a critical step during the manufacture of the Ras protein. After the Ras protein is made in a cell, it must have a fatty molecule attached to it before

it is functional; these drugs (called farnesyl transferase inhibitors) block
that attachment (Barinaga, 1997b). They can also block proteins other
than Ras which seem to be important for cancer cell growth. Farnesyl
transferase inhibitors have been tried in animal models of cancer, and on
cancer cells growing in the laboratory (Barinaga, 1997b). Several have
entered or are about to enter testing in humans (Barinaga, 1997b).

Other oncogenes

It would be a very long and involved process, to list all of the oncogenes
that have been discovered - and no doubt the list would be out of date by
the time that it was written. There are oncogenes involved in every aspect
of cell growth and movement. We have mentioned some that are involved
in the cell cycle, internal signaling and development. There are many
others, including genes such as *fos* and *jun*, which directly regulate DNA.
More are being discovered daily.

The more commonly known oncogenes are listed in Table 4.1 on the
following page.

Table 4.1

Oncogene	Specific role in the cell
Oncogenes which control the cell cycle Bcl 1 Cdk4 Many others suspected	 * Gene for cyclin D1, helps to control the cell cycle * Cyclin-dependant kinases, helps to control the cell cycle
Oncogenes which are growth factor receptors ErB HER-2/neu/erB-2 fms c-kit sis ks/hst int 2	 * receptor for Epidermal Growth Factor * related to the Epidermal Growth Factor Receptor, probably also a growth factor receptor * receptor for Colony Stimulating Factor-1, a growth factor for blood cells * receptor for Stem Cell Factor, a growth factor for melanocytes and some blood cells * part of Platelet Derived Growth Factor * related to Fibroblast Growth Factor * related to Fibroblast Growth Factor
Oncogenes involved in internal signaling Ras, fps, raf, src, abl	 * transmit messages from one part of the cell to another, deliver messages sent from other cells
Oncogenes which turn genes on or Off jun, fos, myc	 * turn genes on and off directly

Chapter 5

Tumor suppressor genes, the good guys

Tumor suppressor genes, as their name implies, prevent cancer. The difference between an oncogene and a tumor suppressor gene might, at first, seem subtle. When a gene mutates to form an oncogene, the resulting abnormal protein stimulates uncontrolled growth. When a tumor suppressor gene mutates, however, its ability to prevent uncontrolled growth is turned off. Normal tumor suppressor genes block cancers in a variety of ways, but many are involved in cell cycle checkpoints. Most cancers have mutations which turn off one or more tumor suppressor genes (Barinaga, 1997b).

Tumor suppressor genes, heredity, and cancer risk

Some families run an increased risk of getting some types of cancers. Usually, such risks are due to mutations in tumor suppressor genes rather than to oncogenes (Fearon, 1997). To understand how the risk increases, it is important to remember that vital genes come in identical pairs. For most tumor suppressors, both tumor suppressor genes in a cell must be damaged in order to promote cancer. In some families, one copy of a particular tumor suppressor gene has already been mutated and is being passed from generation to generation. If a second mutation knocks out the other copy of that tumor suppressor, the cancer can develop (Figure 5.1). For example, mutations in a tumor suppressor gene known as the retinoblastoma gene (or *RB*) result in a cancer of the eye (retinoblastoma) in children. In some families, one copy of the *RB* gene is already nonfunctional; a child who is unlucky enough to get a mutation in the other *RB* gene will develop retinoblastoma. Children from most families, however, are born with 2 normal copies of the *RB* gene and must damage both good copies before the cancer can develop. Children in a family which carries a mutated copy of the *RB* gene will, therefore, be more likely to get retinoblastoma than children in a family who passes down two normal *RB* genes.

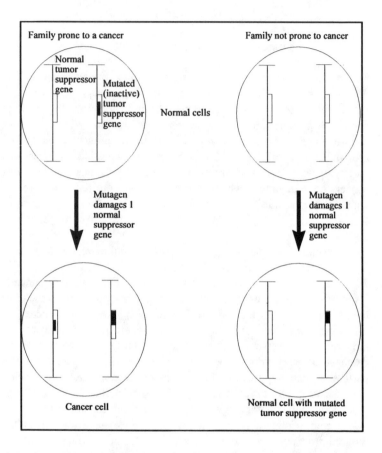

Figure 5.1. A person who inherits a defective tumor suppressor gene is more likely to develop cancer.

A number of tumor suppressor genes, including these shown in Table 5.1, have been discovered recently. We will discuss only a few.

Tumor Suppressor Gene	Associated Cancers
p53	Sarcomas, breast cancer
RB	Retinoblastoma - cancer of the retina of the eye - and other cancers
APC	Colon cancer
DCP4	Cancer of the pancreas
PTCH	Basal cell carcinoma, a skin cancer
BRCA1, BRCA2	Breast cancer

Table 5.1.

P53 and its collaborators stop the cell cycle

Many of the tumor suppressor genes are active in cell cycle checkpoints, controlling either the cyclins or the cell cycle kinases (Marx, 1994). One of the most important of these tumor suppressors has the unassuming name *p53*. Damage to *p53* is very common in cancer cells. The *p53* gene has, in fact, been inactivated in about half of known cancers (Marx, 1994; Levine, 1997). The normal role of the *p53* protein (Figure 5.2) is to sense damage to DNA and shut down the cell cycle until that damage has been repaired (Marx, 1994; Barinaga, 1997b). Cells with mutated genes but an intact *p53* gene are, therefore, prevented from passing on mutations to daughter cells. If the damage cannot be repaired, *p53* turns on a set of proteins which kills the cell. Essentially, if the defective cell is unable to repair its genes, it conveniently commits suicide. This process, known as cell suicide, or apoptosis is a common failsafe in normal cells (Dickman,1997). By inactivating *p53*, cancer cells avoid being killed by their mutations.

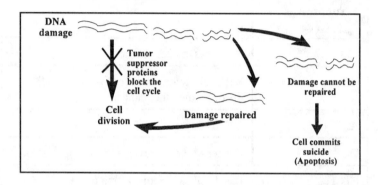

Figure 5.2. When tumor suppressor genes such as p53 sense DNA damage, they stop the cell cycle to allow DNA repair, or trigger cell suicide if the damage is too extensive.

Cancers which don't have *p53* mutations probably contain mutations in other genes of the cell cycle checkpoints (Marx, 1994; Levine, 1997). For instance, the retinoblastoma (*RB*) and *p16* genes aid *p53* in shutting down the cell cycle after DNA damage. Damage to the *RB* gene is associated with several cancers in adults, as well as childhood eye tumors. *P16* is mutated in some melanomas and other cancers (Barinaga, 1997b). Tumors with mutations in *p53* and its partners often respond poorly to treatment; when we discuss apoptosis in chapter 21, we will see why (Levine, 1997). Although *p53* and *RB* are important in cancer formation, damaging them doesn't seem to cause cancer unless other genes are also damaged (Levine, 1997). Damage to the checkpoint genes does, however, allow cells with mutations to survive and divide, and perhaps gives them a longer life span to accumulate damage. Such failure in normal checkpoints may then allow a mutation in an oncogene to slip by, and let the cell start down the path to cancer.

Other tumor suppressor genes don't seem to be directly involved in the cell cycle; instead, they seem to increase the chance that a cell will develop a mutation that turns a gene into an oncogene. These tumor suppressors include such genes as the "breast cancer genes," *BRCA1* and *BRCA2*.

The breast cancer genes

As many as 80% of women who inherit mutations in *BRCA1* or *BRCA2* will develop breast cancer (Marx, 1997). But for a long time, it has been a mystery what these two genes actually do. Now Allan Bradley, Paul Hasty, David Livingstone and their colleagues seem to have finally found a solution. They discovered that normal *BRCA1* and *BRCA2* seem to be important in DNA repair (Marx, 1997). They took mouse cells, damaged the *BRCA2* genes, then exposed the cells to radiation. The cells missing the *BRCA* genes could not repair DNA after radiation damage. Normal mouse cells, however, could. They also discovered that the *BRCA* genes can attach to one of the DNA repair proteins (Marx, 1997). By reducing the cell's ability to repair DNA damage, it seems, the *BRCA* genes increase the chance of a mutation which could lead to cancer.

Other tumor suppressor genes

There are a number of other tumor suppressor genes, as well, which act in a wide variety of ways. Often, their functions are not yet known, but only hinted at. The *FHIT* gene, for example, is missing in a variety of cancers, including colon, breast and lung cancers (Pennisi, 1996c). Some researchers think that *FHIT* may break down a protein that stimulates cell division. One interesting thing about the *FHIT* gene is that it is located at a point on chromosome 3 called a fragile site (Pennisi, 1997). Such fragile sites can be found throughout the chromosomes; they are simply spots that tend to break easily from chemical or other damage. Any gene at a fragile site is particularly likely to be damaged or lost. Researchers may have, in fact, found the actual cause of damage to the *FHIT* gene in one cancer they examined: at the fragile site where *FHIT* is ordinarily found, they instead found genes belonging to a virus.

The *APC* gene is involved in colon cancer. *APC* stands for "adenomatous polyposis coli"; families unfortunate enough to carry mutated copies of this gene tend to develop polyps (small growths) in the colon (Peifer, 1997). Although the polyps themselves are benign, colon cancers often develop within them. Another gene, *DCP4*, is lost or mutated in half of all pancreatic cancers, and possibly in other types of cancer (O'Brien, 1996). Its exact function is not known; however, it may be part of a pathway which inhibits cell growth. Some tumor suppressor genes are little more than names yet. For example, a new tumor suppressor gene known as *PTCH* appears to be a tumor suppressor in basal cell carcinoma, a fairly common skin cancer (Pennisi, 1996b).

How a cancer cell becomes immortal

The genetic changes we've discussed above help to make cancers divide repeatedly. We have not yet, however, discussed any which give a cell immortality. *P53* and *RB* mutations can prolong a cell's life, but the cells still eventually die (Levine, 1997). Why don't cancer cells die like normal cells after a certain number of divisions? Until very recently, no one knew. New discoveries about telomerases and an "immortality gene" may give us some clues.

Telomerases

Telomerases, enzymes which prevent the chromosomes from shortening during cell division, have been hot news in cancer research. These enzymes copy the DNA in the "telomeres," the ends of chromosomes. (Other enzymes duplicate the middle of the chromosome). Without telomerase, a cell's chromosomes shorten each time it copies its genes for cell division. (Luckily, the telomeres do not contain genes and are instead made up of repetitious bits of DNA, so this is not quite as drastic as it at first seems.) The first bit of excitement came when researchers discovered that telomerases are much less active in normal cells than in cancer cells (de Lange, 1998). Some scientists proposed that as normal cells age, the telomeres shorten, resulting in the eventual death of the cell. In cancer cells, on the other hand, telomerases might keep the chromosomes from shortening and prevent the cells from dying. This idea also suggested a possible new cancer treatment. If telomerase is essential to maintain a cancer cell's immortality, then suppressing telomerases may allow the cancer cell to eventually die.

Then a new experiment squelched the excitement. M.A. Blasco and colleagues looked at mice which did not have telomerases (Kelner, 1997). They found that, in fact, the chromosomes did shorten with every cell division (although the mice have survived to at least six generations so far), and they found a large number of abnormalities in the chromosomes. Contrary to expectations, however, the cells from these mice were perfectly capable of forming tumors. The authors suggested that the high telomerase activity in cancers was a meaningless accident. Suddenly, inhibiting telomerases didn't look very promising as a cancer treatment. Nevertheless, doubt remained. What if there were other ways to maintain telomerases in cancer cells in the mutant mice? What if cancers in mice are just different from cancers in humans? Now, a simple new experiment seems to have had the last word in the controversy. A.G. Bodnar and colleagues put telomerase into human cells and examined what happened to the cells (de Lange, 1998). The normal cells died as scheduled (after a predictable number of cell divisions). The cells with telomerases, however, artificially elongated their chromosomes and continued to divide well past their scheduled time of death. These cells looked healthy and vigorous for at least 20 cell divisions beyond the time that the normal cells stopped dividing and began to die. (They did not, however, turn into cancer cells.) Researchers now speculate that the slow shortening of chromosomes in normal human cells may be a built-in mechanism to stop abnormal cells from continuing to divide and turn into cancers. Human cancer cells, it seems, may indeed need to turn on telomerases to prevent chromosome shortening from killing them. Mouse cancers may not. Once again, researchers have been reminded that mice are not humans!

An immortality gene - the first of many?

A new gene may be connected even more closely to cell immortality. Mutations which destroy this gene, called *MORF4* (for "mortality factor from chromosome 4") can give cells the ability to divide forever (Ehrenstein, 1998). Normal *MORF4* keeps cells mortal; if it is added to some cancer cells, they die. *MORF4* acts like a tumor suppressor gene: it takes two bad copies of the gene before a cell becomes immortal.

The structure of *MORF4* makes researchers think that it is a gene which controls other genes. Its levels seem to change in harmony with the cell's stage of life. In young, actively dividing cells, the gene is not very active. As cells slow down and stop dividing, the amount of MORF4 in the cell increases. Defective *MORF4* has been found in some brain cancers, cervical cancer cells and other types of cancers. It is not, however, the only immortality gene. When researchers added *MORF4* to some immortal cells, they became mortal again; however, when they added *MORF4* to other immortal cells, nothing happened. Researchers hope to find the immortality genes in these cells, as well.

To summarize...

In the last two chapters, we have encountered a bewildering number of genes. Any individual cancer will, however, contain only some of these oncogenes and tumor suppressor genes. Nevertheless, the general pattern of mutations leading to cancer is probably similar in all cancers. Initiation occurs when a mutation in one gene, perhaps a cyclin, cyclin-dependent kinases, growth factor, or a member of the internal signaling pathways, turns it into an oncogene. Perhaps a DNA repair enzyme cannot function properly because *BRCA1* or *BRCA2* have been damaged; this could help to increase the chance of such damage. This mutated cell may remain quiet for years. Then promotion occurs when a second mutation occurs or environmental signals send strong growth-promoting signals to the cell. One or more of the proteins which control cell cycle checkpoints (such as *p53*) is also probably inactivated, to allow the cell to divide unchecked. It also seems likely that an immortality gene (such as *MORF4*) also mutates, and that telomerases become more active.

Some types of cancers seem to have stereotypical patterns of change in their genes. For example, colon cancers often start with a mutation in *APC*, followed by mutations in the *Ras* gene, then a gene called *DCC* and finally *p53* (Levine, 1997). In skin cancers, in contrast, the *p53* mutation occurs early, within a different pattern of changes (Levine, 1997). In other cancers, the pattern is again different.

All of these changes in the cell's genes drive the changes in the cell's behavior. They allow the cell to divide uncontrollably. They give it immortality. They allow the expanding mass of cells to invade boundaries of the body that normal cells would not cross. Other genetic changes stimulate the formation of blood vessels to bring more nutrients to enhance their growth. Finally, if the cells change enough, they may become able to enter blood vessels and lymphatic channels and undergo metastasis.

The practical implications of our knowledge of cancer genes

All of this discussion of genes might seem pretty esoteric at the moment. "How does it contribute to cancer treatment?," you might wonder. There are, however, some very practical reasons to know about specific mutations in cancers.

Specific knowledge about cancer genes can give researchers clues about how to treat some cancers. For example, the discovery that the *BRCA* genes are involved in DNA repair suggests that breast cancers with mutated *BRCA* genes might be especially susceptible to radiation treatment. Those breast cancers with *p53* mutations, on the other hand, may be particularly resistant to radiation therapy. If a patient's tumor could be screened for these two mutations, then it might become easier to choose an effective treatment for a particular cancer. Knowledge about oncogenes is also being used to find new types of cancer treatment. In chapter 14, we will discuss how researchers are suppressing abnormal growth factors to slow tumor growth. In chapter 28, we will even see some attempts to directly replace tumor suppressor genes in cancer cells which lack them, or to directly deactivate oncogenes within cancer cells.

Finally, oncogenes and tumor suppressor genes can also help physicians detect people who are at a particularly high risk for some cancers. These people can then be more closely monitored, or given options for preventative treatments. For example, an oncogene called *ret* has been associated with a particularly nasty type of thyroid cancer which runs in some families (Holtzman, 1997). Before the discovery of *ret*, children at risk for this cancer had to undergo frequent screening for thyroid cancer, in the hope of catching it in the early stages. Since the discovery of *ret*, however, children in these families can be tested for the abnormal form of the gene. If it is absent, they may skip the screenings and the worry. If it is present, the thyroid gland can be removed and hormone replacement given, eliminating the chance of getting this deadly disease.

Chapter 6

Traditional cancer treatments - surgery, radiation, and chemotherapy - and how they are changing

Cancer treatments. Some are old, some new. Some are quite safe; others almost as dangerous as the disease. In the rest of the book, we will look at those treatments. Keep in mind, as you read, that many treatments we discuss are experimental and are not yet available to cancer patients in general. Some of these treatments will pass clinical trials (discussed in chapter 8) and eventually become available. Others will turn out to be too dangerous, or not effective enough, in humans, and will fall by the wayside.

The mainstays of cancer therapy for some time have been surgery, radiation, and chemotherapy (treatment with drugs). Not all cancers can be effectively treated with all three; some cancers are sensitive to some types of treatment but not to others. Often, cancer treatments are used in combination. For example, surgery might be used to reduce the size of the tumor, followed by chemotherapy to kill the remaining cancer cells. Radiation and chemotherapy, or radiation and surgery, are combined for other types of tumors. A physician must choose a treatment based on the type of tumor, on how far the tumor cells are believed to have spread, and sometimes, on how aggressive this particular tumor is expected to be in this particular patient.

There are also other, newer treatments, including anti-hormone therapies, vitamins and related chemicals, treatments which boost the immune system, gene therapy, and many others. These are sometimes called adjuvant therapies. Most of them are used in combination with more conventional therapies. In the remainder of the book, we will look at cancer treatments. Our focus will be mainly on the new: on the exciting discoveries and the new frontiers. But, first, we will examine the older treatments, still the mainstays of cancer therapy: surgery, radiation, and traditional chemotherapy. We will look at how they are changing. We will see why they are still so terribly important - and also why it is so terribly important to find additional, new ways to treat some cancers.

Surgery

Surgery is probably the oldest cancer treatment, but it is still one of the most important ones in use today. Despite all of the new technologies such as cryosurgery (freezing) and laser surgery, the principle of surgery is still the same: cut out all of the abnormal cells, and the cancer will be gone. For surgery to be successful as the sole treatment for a cancer, however, all of the cancer cells must be removed; any cell left behind in the body has the potential to redevelop into the same tumor. This is not as easy as it seems, even with isolated tumors that have not metastasized. Although the main body of a tumor may be obvious, cancer cells have usually migrated beyond the edge of the mass and are interspersed with the normal cells surrounding the cancer. So the surgeon plays it safe: he or she removes the visible mass of the tumor and also a large segment of the surrounding, apparently normal cells (Figure 6.1). In this surrounding section, the physician hopes, are any invading cancer cells. After surgery, the tissue is sent for analysis and examined microscopically. A pathologist looks for the cancer cells: irregular, odd looking cells which are often in the midst of cell division. If the edges of the tissue that has been removed are clear of cancer cells, there is a good chance that all of the tumor cells have been removed.

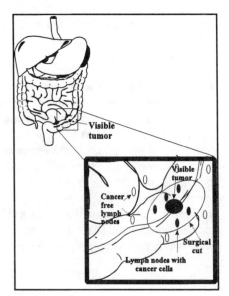

Figure 6.1. During surgery a wide area of tissue around the tumor is removed with the cancer.

Unfortunately, all invading cancer cells may not be detected by their appearance. One problem is that normal organs have all sorts of cells, mixed together, and it can be difficult or even impossible to detect a single cancer cell among them. New technologies are being developed to identify tumor cells by detecting either oncogenes or mutations in tumor suppressor genes (Sidransky, 1997). Some of these studies demonstrate that cancer cells have a sobering tendency to wander far, even in seemingly normal tissues. In recent studies, *p53* mutations were used to identify tumor cells in colon cancers removed during surgery (Sidransky, 1997). In more than half of the patients whose tissue samples looked normal at the edges, tumor cells were detected by the presence of *p53* mutations. In spite of treatment, the cancer returned in approximately a third of these patients, often in the location where the cells with *p53* mutations had been detected. *Ras* mutations could also identify cancer cells in tissues (Sidransky, 1997).

The limitations of surgery

For some tumors, such as a cancer which is confined within the uterus (Look, 1996), or for some early localized skin cancers, surgery alone may result in a cure. For other cancers, however, surgery may be only the first of many treatments. In some cases, the tumor cells have simply spread too far by the time the tumor is detected and the cancer cannot be fully removed. For example, when a tumor has spread throughout the abdominal cavity and has invaded most of the organs, there is little for a surgeon to do except remove as much of the mass as possible without damaging the organs too much. This is sometimes called "debulking". While debulking can alleviate symptoms and reduce the number of tumor cells, it is not a cure. In this situation, surgery is only a preliminary to other therapies. In other cases, where metastasis has occurred, surgical cure is also impossible. A surgeon can remove the original tumor and possibly some of the visible metastasis, but hundreds more may be lying throughout the body. These metastasis can be no more than small undetectable clumps of cells, often in particularly inaccessible organs such as the lungs, the brain, and the liver (See figure 6.2). Against these, the scalpel is of little use.

Figure 6.2 is an endoscopic photograph of metastasis to the liver from the colon. Each nodule is a cancerous growth, which had grown to the point of being inoperable when it was discovered.

Finally, even for cancers which look localized, surgery is often followed by other types of treatments. The recent studies detecting tumor cells by *Ras* and *p53* mutations in colon cancers demonstrate how easy it is to miss tumor cells. Small metastasis outside the tumor area may be missed even more easily. Until a group of tumor cells grows to a certain size, detection is very difficult; technologies such as x-rays cannot detect very small metastasis. In these cases, surgery is used to remove the main mass of cells, and other forms of treatment are used to kill the tumor cells which have not necessarily been detected, but which are suspected to be there.

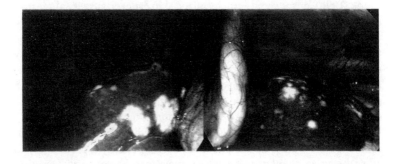

Figure 6.2. photo of liver metastasis.

Chapter 7

Radiotherapy

One of the therapies often combined with surgery is radiation treatment, also called radiotherapy. Over half of all cancer patients receive radiotherapy (Tobias, 1996). Radiation, to many people, is a word that conjures up both fear and mystery. These invisible packets of energy can be so useful, but also so harmful. In its accidental beginnings, however, radiation seemed no more than an innocent toy.

The discovery of x-rays

It was a fall evening in 1895, when Wilhelm Conrad Röntgen, a professor of physics at the University of Wurzberg in Germany accidentally discovered x-rays (Kirz, 1995). He was doing some research in his darkened laboratory, studying beams of electrons from a cathode tube. But when he turned the cathode tube on, some materials left lying about on a bench, some distance away from the tube, lit up. He must have been quite startled! Roentgen discovered that this new technology could be used to see much that was hidden inside the human body. His x-ray of his wife's hand was the first x-ray ever made. Röntgen called his discovery x-rays (although much of the world still calls them Röntgen rays).

Ignorant of the harm that x-rays might cause, people at first used this new technology with abandon. Some people still remember when radiation was used to measure the fit of children's shoes. The harmful effects of x-rays soon became apparent, however, as people who had used x-rays carelessly became injured. But the benefits were quickly apparent, as well. E.H. Gruble made the first attempt to treat cancer with x-rays within a year of Röntgen's discovery. Since that time, radiation therapy has developed into one of the most important treatments for cancer.

How radiation treatment works

Radiotherapy basically works by bombarding the cancer with very energetic particles such as x-rays or gamma rays. The energy is absorbed by cells, and can split water molecules in the cell, producing "free radicals" (Cheville, 1993). Free radicals are very unstable molecules which have temporarily captured an extra electron. This extra electron gives a free radical the ability to combine with any other molecule nearby. The free radicals bounce around in the cell, wreaking havoc as they damage critical molecules. DNA damage can be particularly fatal. For a long time, in fact, researchers believed that it was DNA damage that directly killed the cancer cells. Recent experiments, however, suggest that the DNA damage may be only part of the story. Radiation therapy may, in fact, need to trigger apoptosis (cell suicide) to be fully effective (Corvio, 1996). As you may recall from chapter 5, apoptosis is the cell's response to excessive DNA damage which cannot be repaired. As you may also remember, some cancer cells have mutations in the genes which trigger apoptosis, such as p53, and do not die in spite of severe damage to their DNA. These new findings may explain why radiotherapy is not effective for some cancers. Some researchers suggest screening patients for p53 mutations, to determine who might or might not be a good candidate for radiotherapy (Corvio, 1996).

Like surgery, radiation has its limitations. In most cases it is of little use in metastasis. Whole body radiation would as likely kill as cure, if it were set to levels which could penetrate all internal organs to unknown sites of metastasis. In addition, some types of tumors are just not very sensitive to radiation. For other tumors, however, it is a very effective and common form of cancer treatment.

External radiotherapy

The two basic forms of radiotherapy are external beam radiotherapy and internal radiotherapy (Figure 7.1). In external beam therapy, sophisticated machines produce high energy particles outside the body and focus them on the site of the cancer. Both high energy x-rays and gamma rays have traditionally been used. X-rays are very energetic particles of light which are made when a normal atom is hit with a burst of energy. Gamma rays are similar particles spontaneously given off when certain radioactive elements (such as radium, uranium, and cobalt) decay. X-rays and gamma rays do not distinguish between normal cells and cancer cells; any cell they hit can be damaged. Normal cells can, however, be spared by choosing radiation doses carefully and focusing the beam precisely. Recent advances have made such focusing extraordinarily precise. With complex calculations and multiple beams from different directions, radiation can now match even the shape of the tumor (Brahme, 1996).

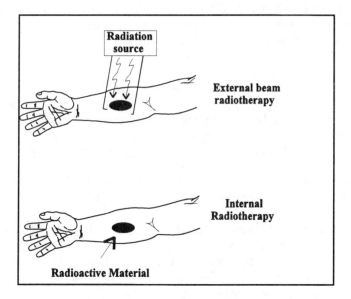

Figure 7.1. Comparison of external beam and internal radiotherapy.

Researchers are also finding ways to use other types of high energy particles for cancer treatment. In Japan, an expensive new machine, the Heavy Ion Medical Accelerator (HIMAC) produces beams of carbon ions (Nomile, 1997). These charged carbon atoms can be focused more tightly than x-rays, with less damage to surrounding normal tissues. Their larger size and charge can also produce more injury to the tumor.

High doses of radiation have been given with this accelerator, with good responses, and apparently no serious side effects so far (although some researchers caution that long-term side effects from such high doses may not show up until 3 or 4 years after treatment). More than 100 patients have been treated with radiation from the new accelerator and at least half of them have responded to the treatment. All of these patients had untreatable tumors or tumors that were resistant to conventional radiation treatment. HIMAC is, to this date, the world's only heavy ion accelerator. A major reason is the expense. It cost $326 million to build and $58 million a year to operate! U.S. scientists are hoping that beams of protons, the positively charged particles from the centers of atoms, will have the same benefits as carbon ions. Accelerators for protons are less powerful and are, therefore, cheaper to build and operate.

Internal radiotherapy

If the tumor is easily accessible, radiation treatments may also be given by temporarily placing small amounts of radioactive material directly in the tumor; this is called internal radiotherapy or brachytherapy. The radioactive materials are enclosed in small rods or other devices that allow them to be easily removed at the end of the treatment. Internal radiotherapy is very common for some cancers such as cervical cancers.

An alternative, for some types of cancers, is to inject a radioactive material into the blood which carries it to the site of the cancer. This treatment can kill tumors which are too far from body surfaces to easily place and remove radioactive materials. In this case, however, the radioactive material must be very carefully chosen. It must find its way to the cancer and not be taken up elsewhere in the body. For example, radioactive iodine is sometimes used to treat thyroid gland tumors (Berkow, 1992). The thyroid gland is the only place in the body where iodine is taken up from the blood and concentrated in significant amounts.

Radioactive iodine in the blood will enter the thyroid cancer cells and kill them, without harming other organs. One limitation on this type of internal radiotherapy is that the radioactive material must quickly decay to become non-radioactive; it cannot be removed like other forms of internal radiotherapy.

Unfortunately, natural radioactive compounds which find their way to tumors are relatively rare. Cancer researchers are, however, trying to make artificial radioactive drugs which do the same thing. One possibility is to attach radioactive atoms to guidance molecules which will seek out cancer cells. Antibodies, for example, can carry radioactive molecules to tumors. We will discuss these hybrid molecules, known as immunotoxins, or "magic bullets" in chapter 11.

Side effects

Radiation treatment has more side effects than surgery. It can damage normal cells, in particular those which are rapidly dividing and in the path of the radiation. Radiotherapy often results in fatigue, and sometimes in red and irritated skin, at the site where the radiation is being given. Other side effects may be seen, depending in the area of the body which is being irradiated. For example, when the abdomen is irradiated, patients can have nausea and other intestinal upsets. Radiation can also damage the cells in the bone marrow which make blood cells. The resulting decreases in blood cells can cause tiredness from low oxygen levels in the blood, bleeding from abnormal blood clotting, and an increased susceptibility to infections.

Taking into account an individual's sensitivity to radiation

One interesting new concept in radiation therapy is based on the observation that the same levels of radiation can affect individuals very differently (Peters, 1996; Burner, 1996). The dose that severely damages the normal cells of one person may have much less effect on the cells of another. "Safe" levels of radiation are based on the average sensitivity in the population (Peters, 1996). If individual variability could, however, be exploited, then radiation doses could be more closely tailored to the specific person undergoing radiotherapy (Figure 7.2). A person whose normal cells are less sensitive than average might be able to get higher doses of radiation, with a better chance of killing the tumor cells , but without risking a dangerous increase in the side effects. A person with a particularly high sensitivity to radiation could be given lower doses to decrease side effects, or perhaps given an alternative form of treatment.

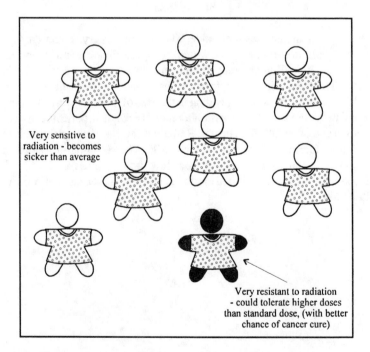

Very sensitive to radiation - becomes sicker than average

Very resistant to radiation - could tolerate higher doses than standard dose, (with better chance of cancer cure)

Figure 7.2. Individual susceptibility to radiation varies.

The problem is, of course, how to predict the sensitivity of an individual before he or she has been exposed to radiation. Some researchers have found that fibroblasts, a common cell in the skin, can be used to predict the radiation sensitivity of normal tissues (Peters, 1996). If, for example, a person's fibroblasts are severely damaged by a particular dose of radiation, then he or she is expected to have severe side effects from radiation treatment. Several technical problems must still be overcome before this test can become practical (Figure 7.3). Nevertheless, the day may not be too far off when skin samples are collected from every person before radiotherapy, and used to calculate an individual dose of radiation for that person.

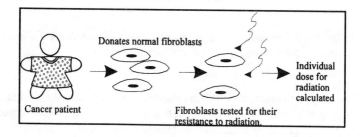

Donates normal fibroblasts

Cancer patient

Fibroblasts tested for their resistance to radiation.

Individual dose for radiation calculated

Figure 7.3. Susceptibility to radiation can be tested by irradiating normal cells such as skin fibroblasts.

Resistance to radiation and the use of radiosensitizers

For a variety of reasons, radiotherapy does not always work. Chemicals called radiosensitizers may, however, make tumors more sensitive to radiation. Sometimes, radiotherapy fails because some tumors have too little oxygen in some areas (D.J. Lee, 1996). Oxygen prolongs the life of the free radicals made from water by radiation (Berkow, 1992). It also allows cells to grow more rapidly; dividing cells are most susceptible to radiotherapy. As a tumor grows, however, the tumor cells may grow faster than the new blood vessels which bring oxygen. As a consequence, cancer cells can become resistant to radiation (Figure 7.4).

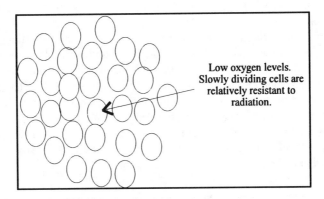

Figure 7.4. Many tumors contain areas where oxygen levels are low and the
tumor cells are resistant to some treatments.

One way to counteract radiation resistance is to increase the amount of
oxygen in a tumor. For example, patients may sometimes breathe gases
high in oxygen before radiation therapy (Teicher, 1994). One possibility
is hyperbaric oxygen, pure (100%) oxygen at a higher than normal
pressure (Berkow, 1992; D.J. Lee, 1996). (Normal air, incidentally,
contains 21 % oxygen.) Carbogen, an alternative, is a mixture of 95 %
oxygen and 5% carbon dioxide (Teicher, 1994). Mice breathing carbogen
have been cured with lower doses of radiation than without carbogen
(Ono, 1994). In humans, the results have been less clear-cut, but some
benefits have been seen. For example, in one recent study, carbogen
increased the response of bladder cancers to radiation (Hoskin, 1997).
The numbers of patients enrolled in this study were small; therefore, the
authors suggest that results are promising, but need to be confirmed with
larger numbers of people.

A different way to counteract the effects of low oxygen is to replace
oxygen with other chemicals which can prolong the life of free radicals.
For example, nitroimidazoles may be able to make some cancers more
sensitive to radiotherapy (D.J. Lee, 1996). Researchers are also excited
about the possibilities of some new chemicals, the Texaphyrins.

Texaphyrins - everything is bigger in Texas

Texaphyrins are members of a group of chemicals known as porphyrins. Porphyrins, which look a bit like a 4 leaf clover (Adams, 1998), are very useful molecules in the human body. (Among other duties, they carry oxygen and iron in the blood.) Porphyrins also tend to accumulate in cancer cells and not in normal cells. This characteristic has made them very important in a treatment called phototherapy, discussed in chapter 19. Texaphyrin is a new, bigger "5-leaved" porphyrin which may be useful for both phototherapy and radiation treatment (Pharmacyclics, 1997; Adams, 1998).

Texaphyrin is the brainchild of Jonathan Sessler, a chemist at the University of Texas, Austin (Adams, 1998). For the last 14 years, Sessler has been trying to make a bigger porphyrin; he hoped that such a molecule might be able to carry cancer drugs or other big molecules into a cancer cell with it. He finally succeeded, with Texaphyrin. (On a lighter note, Sessler admits to an ulterior motive for making a bigger porphyrin: state pride. "Everything is bigger in Texas", he quipped, in an interview in the scientific journal Science (Adams, 1998)). Texaphyrin is usually attached to a variety of metal atoms, including gadolinium, cadmium, and lutetium (Adams, 1998; Pharmacyclics, 1997). Some of these forms of Texaphyrin may be useful as radiosensitizers. (Adams, 1998; Pharmacyclics, 1997). For example, when Texaphyrin is attached to gadolinium, it seems to make nearby free radicals last longer (Adams, 1998). In mice, gadolinium Texaphyrin has been able to make radiation treatment more effective (Adams, 1998). It has been recently tried in cancer patients with metastasis to the brain (Carde, 1997). At the American Society of Clinical Oncology meeting in 1997, researchers reported that, so far, there has been no substantial side effects from this treatment (Carde, 1997). Data were available on 6 patients: tumors had completely disappeared in two patients, shrunk in three patients, and stopped growing in one.

Other ways to make a cell more sensitive to radiation

There are also other ways to make cancer cells more sensitive to radiation. One is to give them drugs which prevent them from repairing DNA damage after radiation treatment. Hydroxyurea, for example, prevents DNA bases from being made (McGinn, 1996). It has been used as a radiosensitizer for many different types of cancers. Unfortunately, it is difficult to detect whether hydroxyurea has any clear benefit in many studies, because patients have been given many different drugs at the same time (McGinn, 1996). In some studies of cervical cancer, however, it did seem to show a clear cut benefit, compared to radiation alone (McGinn, 1996). Some new drugs, such as Fludarabine, may also prevent the repair of DNA damage (McGinn, 1996). Another new drug, an artificial sugar called 2-deoxy-D-glucose (2DG), seems to simply compete with normal blood sugar (glucose) and reduce the amount of energy available to a cell (Mohanti, 1996). Since energy is needed for any manufacturing process in the cell, this can also decrease DNA repair. 2DG has shown promise in cancer tests in animals (Mohanti, 1996). It has recently been shown to be safe in human patients with brain tumors (Mohanti, 1996).

Bromodeoxyuridine and iododeoxyuridine are drugs that have been used as radiosensitizers in a number of different cancers (McGinn, 1996). These drugs, called thymine analogues, look like the DNA base thymine and are used like thymine to make new DNA - but their presence makes the new strand of DNA particularly fragile. The strand becomes susceptible to breaks from radiation wherever these molecules have been incorporated instead of real thymine. Other drugs, such as 5-fluorouracil, may drive the cancer cell into stages of the cell cycle which are particularly sensitive to radiation (McGinn, 1996).

Gene therapy and radiation sensitization

Some researchers hope to eventually deliver radiosensitizing genes instead of drugs to cancer cells. These genes would be turned on by radiation, and produce proteins which either make the cancer cell more sensitive to the effects of radiation, or which directly kill the cell (Buschbaum, 1996). The process is illustrated in figure 7.5.

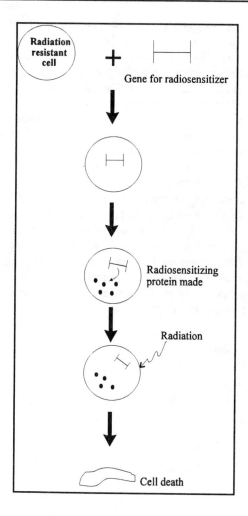

Figure 7.5. Genes for radiosensitizers can be put into cells, making them more sensitive to radiation.

Exploiting low oxygen levels, instead of preventing them

A great deal of effort has been expended to find drugs and other treatments which can reverse the effects of low oxygen concentration in tumors during radiation therapy. Some researchers, however, look on low oxygen levels as an opportunity, instead of a problem. Their idea is to not modify the oxygen concentration, but to exploit it. They suggest using drugs which are not dangerous in tissues with normal levels of oxygen, but which become deadly when they are in low oxygen environments (D.J. Lee, 1996). These drugs are sometimes called the "hypoxic Cytotoxins" (which basically means "low oxygen cell killers"). One example of these drugs is tirapazamine (or SR 4233) (D.J. Lee, 1996; Brown, 1994). Tirapazamine is 40 to 150 times more lethal to cells in low-oxygen environments than to normal cells. When it is deprived of oxygen, tirapazamine loses an electron, which forms free radicals. The free radicals then damage and kill the cell. A similar drug, RSU 1069, also appears to be an effective killer of cancer cells (Brown, 1994). Such drugs may be particularly useful when they are combined with treatments that kill well-oxygenated cells, such as radiotherapy.

Chapter 8

The search for new drugs

Chemotherapy is the treatment of cancer with drugs. It is the only one of the three traditional therapies - surgery, radiation, chemotherapy - which is usually useful for metastatic cancer. Chemotherapy is big business, with over two dozen companies competing for the profits. Combined annuals sales for the four most commonly used prostate cancer drugs are approximately 1.7 billion dollars (Roush, 1997b). Tamoxifen, used for breast cancer, accounts for $500 million a year, and Paclitaxel (Taxol) $800 million (Roush, 1997b). All over the world, drug companies are competing to discover the next "hot new cancer drug," find their name in headlines across newspapers, and ensure their company's profits. But where do these drugs come from? And how do they get from the laboratory to the pharmacy? In this chapter, we will find out.

Drug development - how new drugs are found

Since the 1950's, thousands of potential anticancer drugs have been found in laboratories throughout the world (Gura, 1997c). Of those thousands, only 39 cancer drugs had been approved by the Federal Drug Administration (Gura, 1997c). The process of drug development, from laboratory to clinic, is long, arduous, and expensive. All new cancer drugs must pass a rigorous set of tests designed to make certain that they are both effective and reasonably safe in humans (Figure 8.1). In preclinical testing, the drug is tested in cancer cells growing outside the body and in animals. A drug which looks promising in preclinical testing is then moved into human clinical trials, where it is tested in volunteers with cancer. It is not rare for this process to take years.

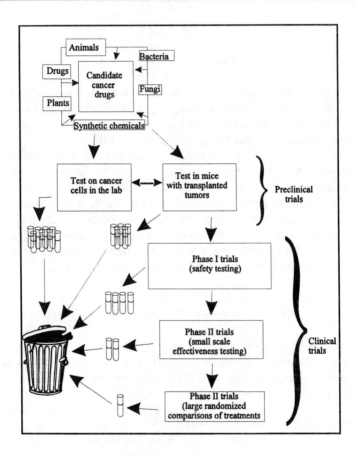

Figure 8.1. The process of testing new cancer drugs.

Where drugs come from

The first step in drug development is, of course, to find something to test. Most new drugs come from screening natural products (Markman, 1997). Many new drugs have come from plants; others are from bacteria, animals such as corals or even from fungi. Many candidate drugs come from mass screenings sponsored by agencies such as the National Cancer Institute. Sometimes, however, they are found just by chance, offshoots of an experiment intended to test something else. Occasionally, drugs prescribed for another disease are found to have cancer fighting ability.

Existing cancer drugs are also modified in the hope of making them more effective or less toxic (Unger, 1996). The newest approach is to design drugs with a specific shape to target tumor suppressor gene or oncogene products (Unger, 1996). This approach, of course, requires an extensive knowledge of how both normal and cancer cells work, and has only become practical with recent advances in that knowledge.

Preclinical testing

Cancer drugs are tested for years, before they are tried in human cancer patients. Potential drugs must first be able to kill cancer cells in the laboratory. These cells may either be cells from patients' tumors which are maintained artificially outside the body, or actual cancers in laboratory animals, usually mice. Both approaches have their advantages - and their drawbacks.

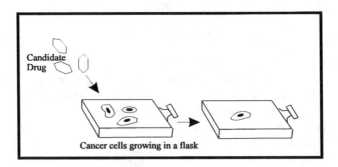

Figure 8.2. Drugs can be tested by adding them to cancer cells in the laboratory.

The easiest and cheapest method to test a cancer drug's effectiveness is to add the drug to cancer cells grown in the laboratory (Figure 8.2), then observe the cells to detect cell death or slowing of their growth (Gura, 1997c). These are known as cell culture tests (shown in Figure 8.1). Many potential cancer drugs have been found in cell culture tests. This approach does, however, have its problems. The biggest problem is that it can't mimic the complexity of the human body. A drug which kills cancer cells may also kill normal body cells, or have other dangerous side effects. Cell culture tests also cannot predict whether the drug can be delivered to the site of the cancer. Not all drugs injected into the body reach all areas of the body. For example, some drugs may be eliminated from the body (usually by the liver and kidneys) too quickly to do any good.

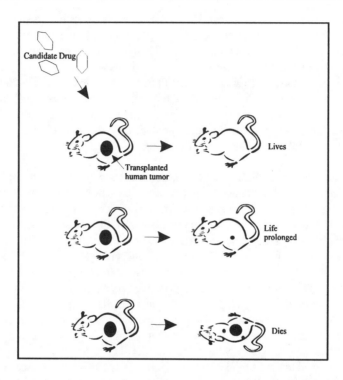

Figure 8.3. Drugs can be tested in mice carrying transplanted human tumors.

The second common screening method is to test the drugs in mice (Figure 8.3) carrying transplanted human tumors (Gura, 1997c). This system may be the best way to mimic what would happen to the drug in the human body (Unger, 1996). The three possible outcomes of such a test are illustrated in Figure 8.3. Theoretically, drug delivery, safety and effectiveness should be similar in mice and humans. Unfortunately, this assumption is not always true. Mice and other test animals sometimes seem to handle drugs differently than the human body (Gura, 1997c). In addition, the transplanted human tumors may behave differently in the mice than they would in humans. For example, some tumors which metastasize in humans don't metastasize in mice (Gura, 1997c). Finally, this system is much more expensive than testing drugs in cell culture. A more expensive test means that fewer drugs will actually get tested.

New evidence also suggests that some effective drugs may actually be missed by screening candidate drugs against transplanted human tumors in mice. Recently, Jacqueline Plowman and her colleagues at the National Cancer Institute tested twelve anti-cancer drugs which are currently used for the treatment of cancer and are known to be effective against some cancers (Gura, 1997c). They found that none of the drugs were effective against 30 of 48 transplanted human tumors in mice. If these drugs had been originally screened by this method, they would likely have been rejected at the very first stages of testing.

Some researchers think that the basic problem with screening drugs in mice is that using human tumors in mice may simply be too unnatural a system. They would like to develop more mice with natural mouse tumors which closely mimic human tumors. Generally, this means breeding mice which have the same oncogenes as humans with that tumor. For example, there are now mice which lack *APC*, the gene which is missing or damaged in humans with a family history of colon cancer (Gura, 1997c). The good news is that these tumors behave very similarly to human colon cancers in their early stages. The bad news is that, in the later stages of disease, the human and mouse colon cancers are very different. Some experiments have been even more discouraging. A set of mice missing the retinoblastoma gene, which should develop eye tumors, instead developed tumors of the pituitary gland (Gura, 1997c). Then there were the mice with the damaged breast cancer gene, *BRCA1*; they developed no tumors at all! (Gura, 1997c).

At the moment, however, there are no better alternatives than the two systems described above - and, in spite of the flaws, new drugs are being found. In fact, researchers are actually finding too many rather than too few potential drugs. The National Cancer Institute has screened approximately 63,000 compounds in the last 7 years, and found 5,000 which are promising as cancer drugs (Gura, 1997c). Most of these 5,000 will turn out not to work in humans, or be too toxic to use. One problem with having so many potential new drugs is choosing which to test further. There is simply not enough money or the facilities to test all of them. For the moment, the National Cancer Institute's solution is to test those first which appear to act differently from the known chemotherapy drugs. In this way, they hope to find unique new drugs, rather than just chemically different versions of currently used drugs (Gura, 1997c).

The drugs that seem promising will be further tested in animals and cancer cells growing in the laboratory. Extensive animal testing must determine that the drug is indeed effective against cancers and appears to be safe. Many drugs do not make it through these tests. Technical problems with administering the drug may also limit their usefulness. After years of initial testing, a few drugs will make it through the tests and move on to testing in humans, called clinical trials.

Clinical trials

There is no guarantee that a drug which was promising in laboratory animals will also work in humans. Too often, new treatments have cured cancer in mice, but failed miserably in humans. Mice and humans are, often, just too different. Therefore, new drugs (and all other new cancer treatments) must be tested in a brave set of human volunteers with cancer, before they are released to cancer patients in general.

Clinical trials of drugs are usually divided into three stages, called phases I, II and III. In the first stage, called phase I, the new drug is tested for safety in a small group of human volunteers with cancer. Usually the volunteers are patients whose cancer cannot be effectively treated with current techniques (National Cancer Institute, 1998d). Small groups of patients are given increasing doses of the drug, to determine how large a dose a person can tolerate without major side effects. From these studies, a dose is determined for the new drug. Generally, Phase I safety studies are not designed to test the effectiveness of the drug - although there is always the hope that the human volunteers will be rewarded for their participation by a cure or a lengthened lifespan. New drugs which are too toxic are not tested further.

Drugs which have successfully passed the safety hurdle usually move into small scale "efficacy" trials, which determine whether the new drug shows promise of effectiveness in human cancer (National Cancer Institute, 1998d). These are called phase II trials. Usually, the volunteers are a group of people with one type of cancer, or closely related types of cancer, who have little hope of cure with conventional treatments. Several tests of the drug, with a total of hundreds of patients, are usually run in phase II trials (phase I trials often have fewer than 100 people). Because such large numbers of patients are usually involved, phase II trials sometimes discover unusual side effects which occur in only a few people.

One difficulty with testing new drugs is finding the hundreds of volunteers needed for clinical trials of each drug. It might seem surprising, at first, that drugs must be tested in such large numbers of people. The large numbers are, however, dictated by an element of chance which always exists in biology. People's bodies (and tumors) vary considerably. As a result, any two individuals will respond a little differently to an identical treatment. Two groups of people will also be a little different. Therefore, simply by the choice of participants in a drug trial, it can look as if a new treatment is more (or less) effective than the old. There is, however, a way to deal with this problem. As the numbers of participants gets larger, variability between groups will diminish. Differences which remain between very large groups of people would, therefore, be expected to be real. The more subtle the response, the more people must be tested to rule out chance.

Finally, the promising drugs from phase II trials move into the last stage of testing. Phase III trials compare the new treatment to the current "state of the art" treatment in large numbers of patients (National Cancer Institute, 1998d). Usually, there are two or more groups of volunteers in these trials. One group, for example, will receive the conventional treatment for their particular type of tumor. The other group will receive the new drug, either alone or as part of their treatment. Cancer patients who enroll in phase III trials are randomly assigned to each group without knowing which treatment they will receive. By comparing the response to treatment in the two groups, researchers can determine whether the new drug should become a standard treatment for a particular cancer and the drug company can apply for FDA approval. It is only after FDA approval has been granted, that drugs become available to cancer patients in general.

Measuring the results of clinical trials -
complete remissions, partial remissions, or stable disease

Although it might seem reasonable to report the results of clinical trials as the number of patients cured by the new treatment, the truth is that cancer is a disease where it is difficult to measure cures. In some patients, the cancer will indeed disappear. But it may come back in a month, or a year, or perhaps longer. In general, the longer the cancer does not return, the greater the likelihood is that it has truly been cured. It is impossible, however, to say that it will never come back. The effectiveness of cancer drugs is, therefore, measured as complete remissions, meaning that the cancer can no longer be detected, or partial remissions, or stable disease (a cancer which has been progressing no longer progresses). Many times, cancer treatments will only produce remissions in a minority of patients. A complete remission rate of 30% for example, might be considered successful for some types of cancer. Another common statistic is the average survival time with the new treatment. With some types of cancers, simply remaining alive longer after treatment may be an important goal. With this background in mind, let's take a look at some of the drugs which have made it through this process, and some others that are in the midst of these tests.

Chapter 9

Tried and true anti-cancer drugs -
and some of their newer relatives

A "cancer drug," these days, can refer to many things. Hidden behind a name that sounds much like any other drug name, you might find a byproduct of a vitamin. Or a drug which suppresses hormones to slow cancer growth. You might even find that the drug is actually an antibody or a cytokine, both products of the immune system. In this book, we will discuss all of these things. But, first, we will look at some very traditional chemotherapy drugs. These are the drugs sometimes called "cytotoxic" drugs, meaning "drugs that kill cells".They are generally not subtle drugs; they are highly toxic to normal cells as well as cancer cells. Usually, they act on rapidly dividing cells; they spare most normal cells simply because normal cells don't divide as often as cancer cells. Their side effects can be nasty; if the dose is accidentally too high, they could kill. But, very often, they are one of the most effective ways to kill cancer cells.

There are dozens of drugs used for cancer treatment; many of them are variations of each other, designed to be more effective or less toxic or better absorbed into the cancer cells. Cancer drugs are, therefore, often discussed as groups of related drugs. If you know how one member of that group works, there is a good chance that its relatives will work much the same.

Drugs which damage cells through their DNA

Most of the currently used cytotoxic drugs damage DNA in some way. They may interfere with DNA synthesis, make the DNA more fragile and easy to break, or prevent it from making its protein.

Alkylating agents, modern descendants of chemical warfare drugs

One large group of DNA damaging drugs, called the alkylating agents, are relatives of chemical warfare weapons developed in World War I and World War II (Salmon, 1987). These drugs transfer chemical groups called alkyl groups to bases in DNA (as well as to other molecules in the cell). Alkylation (Figure 9.1) can create mutations by confusing the enzymes which duplicate or repair DNA, causing them to put the wrong base on the strand across from the alkylated base. Sometimes, enzymes in the cell remove the base with the alkyl group; this can cause breaks in the DNA. One of the most important events in alkylation, however, is when the alkyl groups on two different bases attach to each other and "cross-link" the DNA molecule. This abnormal connection prevents the DNA strands from being pulled apart for DNA duplication or protein production. A number of chemotherapy drugs are alkylating agents: chlorambucil (Leukeran), cyclophosphamide (Cytoxan) and its newer relative ifosfamide, mitomycin (mitomycin C, Mitocin-C, Mutamycin) and many others. The alkylating agents are some of the most commonly used drugs in cancer. Other types of drugs such as Cisplatin (Platinol) and the newer Carboplatin also seem to work partially by alkylation. Since the alkylating drugs have been so useful, but yet very toxic, many are spawning new relatives which are expected to be either safer or more effective (or, preferably, both). For example, Trofosfamide, a new drug related to cyclophosphamide, recently passed phase I (safety) trials (Blomqvist, 1995).

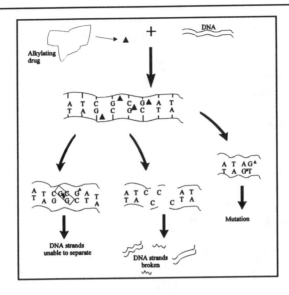

Figure 9.1. Alkylating drugs add alkyl groups to bases in DNA, with three possible outcomes

Cancer drugs, courtesy of bacteria

We often think of bacteria as something scary, or unclean, or something to be avoided at all costs. Some very useful drugs have, however, been found in these much-maligned members of society. Bacteria often make chemicals to defend themselves against other bacteria; many useful antibiotics (drugs which kill bacteria) have been found this way. Some very effective cancer drugs have also come from bacteria, particularly from a group known as *Streptomyces*. For example, one group of these drugs, the anthracyclines, have turned out to be some of the most valuable chemotherapy agents in use today. The oldest members of this group are Doxorubicin (Adriamycin) and daunorubicin (Cerubidine). The anthracyclines insert themselves inside the DNA molecule and block the two strands from separating. This prevents DNA duplication during cell division, and also stops the production of messenger RNA. One serious problem with the anthracyclines is that they can cause irreversible damage to the heart with high doses (Salmon, 1987). Researchers are developing newer anthracyclines (such as epirubicin) which have a decreased risk of damaging the heart (Coukell, 1997).

Drugs which shut down the DNA factory

Other drugs do not damage DNA but, instead, prevent its manufacture (or "synthesis"). DNA synthesis is important in two situations: DNA repair and cell division. During DNA repair, damaged DNA is removed and replaced by new DNA. New DNA is also made during cell division, when chromosomes are made for each new cell.

DNA synthesis is a long and involved process. In a way, however, it resembles the manufacture of any large, complicated piece of equipment. First, the individual parts, or building blocks, must be made - then these pieces must be put together. In the case of DNA, the building blocks are simply the bases - adenine, guanine, cytosine and thymine - carried on individual sugar molecules. After the building blocks are made, different sets of enzymes string them together in the proper order. Various cancer drugs interfere with all of these stages of DNA synthesis (Figure 9.2).

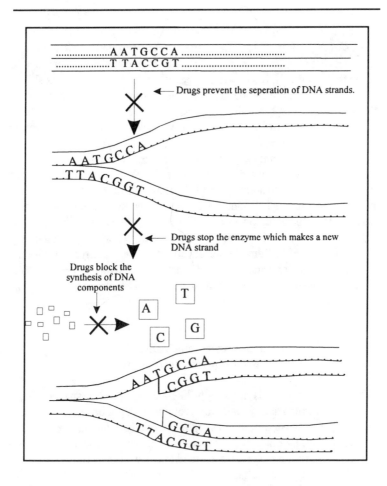

Figure 9.2. Drugs can prevent the manufacture of new DNA in several different ways.

Some of the most effective drugs are those which prevent the building blocks of DNA from ever being made. These drugs don't have to be able to block all of the bases from being made; they can simply block one to stop DNA synthesis. It's as if a factory making cars no longer was able to get a vital part for the engine: it would simply have to stop manufacturing the whole car. For example, 5-fluorouracil (5-FU) stops the cell from making the base thymine (by blocking the enzyme thymidylate synthase, which makes thymine from uracil) (McGinn, 1996). A new relative of 5-FU, ZD1694 (Tomudex), was designed by manipulating chemical structures to make a molecule which would have fewer side effects than 5-FU, but be easier to administer (Takemura, 1997). ZD1694 has looked promising in phase I, II, and III clinical trials against several types of cancer, particularly colon cancer (Takemura, 1997). It seems to be as effective as 5-FU, but less toxic. Several other drugs, including Methotrexate (MTX, amethopterin) and its newer relatives (Takimoto, 1995), 6-mercaptopurine (6-MP, Purinethol) and hydroxyurea (Hydrea) also interfere with enzymes involved in the manufacture of DNA building blocks.

New drugs which block DNA twists -
Topoisomerase Inhibitors

DNA in a living cell is not simply like a long strand of spaghetti. It is twisted and coiled and wound onto proteins. It might be better, in fact, to think of it as a twisted strand of spaghetti wound around little spools. The twists in the DNA are quite important. The twisting makes the DNA molecule more compact (to understand this, try taking a rubber band and twisting it and see what happens to its length and size). Twisting (called "supercoiling" by biologists) also prepares the molecules for processes that require the two DNA strands to be separated, such as duplication of DNA or production of messenger RNA and proteins.

Topoisomerases are enzymes inside the nucleus which twist DNA in the nucleus more tightly, or relax it. As the enzymes which copy DNA or make messenger RNA move along the strands of DNA, topoisomerases keep the twists at the right level; over- or underwinding can inhibit these processes. Topoisomerases break the DNA molecule, untwist or twist it, then rejoin the strands. Topoisomerase inhibitors are one of the newest additions to the cancer drug arsenal.

The first topoisomerase inhibitor, camptothecin, came from the bark of *Camptotheca acuminata*, a tree from China (Research Triangle Institute, 1998). Camptothecin was abandoned 20 years ago, because it was too toxic in clinical trials (Research Triangle Institute, 1998). Now it's back, in a slightly different chemical form. It turns out that some of the problems with the original form may have occurred because the active drug does not dissolve in water. (Incidentally, some unscrupulous souls are advertising "non - prescription" forms of camptothecin, made by soaking the bark in water.) There are also newer relatives of camptothecin, which may be more effective and less toxic: Topotecan and irinotecan are two of these drugs. Topotecan and irinotecan have been active in preclinical studies against various cancers, and have shown some promise for the treatment of breast cancer in phase I (safety) trials (O'Reilly, 1995). Phase II trials using irinotecan in colon cancer have been recently completed and have also been promising (Rougier, 1997). Topoisomerase inhibitors are now being tested in Phase II trials for breast and other cancers (O'Reilly, 1995).

Messing up the microtubules

Another group of drugs kills cancer cells by interfering with microtubules, structures that look like tiny tubes. Microtubules are used in a number of ways in the cell. One of their jobs is to transport molecules from one end of the cell to the other. They are not, however, permanent structures. When a microtubule is needed, it forms out of proteins called tubulins; when its purpose is done, it is broken down into tubulins again. The tubulins are then recycled for the next job. In a normal cell, this goes on constantly. The mitotic spindle is a particularly dramatic example of microtubule assembly and disassembly. It forms in the middle of the cell during cell division. It then sorts the chromosomes, moves one set of chromosomes to one new cell and the other set to the other new cell, then disassembles and allows the two new cells to split apart. Some drugs kill cancer cells by interfering with microtubule formation or breakdown.

From periwinkles to cancer -Vinca alkaloids

The drugs vinblastine (Velban) and Vincristine (Oncovin), known as "vinca alkaloids," come from the periwinkle plant (*Vinca rosea*). They stop tubulin molecules from assembling into microtubules (Berkow, 1992; Salmon, 1987). By preventing the mitotic spindle from forming, they stop cell growth and kill the cell. A cell treated with the Vincristine or vinblastine will be trapped in the middle of cell division, with two sets of chromosomes hopelessly stuck in the middle of the cell. New vinca alkaloids such as vinorelbine (Navelbine) are being tested in clinical trials (O'Reilly, 1995; Goa, 1994). Vinorelbine has fewer side effects, particularly nerve damage, than its relatives (Goa, 1994). It has shown promise in many different types of cancers, including some advanced cases and difficult-to-treat tumors (O'Reilly, 1995; Goa, 1994; Husain, 1994).The most famous drug which interferes with microtubules is not, however, a vinca alkaloid; it is an entirely different kind of drug and is known as Paclitaxel, or Taxol.

Paclitaxel (Taxol) and Docetaxel

In the 1990s, perhaps the hottest new cancer drug has been Paclitaxel (Taxol), which comes from the bark of the Pacific yew tree, *Taxus brevifolia*. Paclitaxel was actually discovered in the 1960's, in a program which screened large numbers of plants for activity against cancer (National Cancer Institute, 1998c). But, as we have seen, it is a very long road from a promising chemical to an FDA approved cancer drug, and there are many drugs competing for attention - so Paclitaxel was shelved for a while. In the late 1970s, however, the discovery of how Paclitaxel works sparked researchers' interest; it seemed to be something unique, and not just another slightly altered version of a chemotherapy drugs already on the market. Since the 1980's, a number of preclinical and clinical trials have demonstrated that Paclitaxel is indeed an effective new drug for the treatment of cancer. It has been approved by the FDA for advanced breast cancer and ovarian cancer and is in clinical trials for a number of other types of cancer (National Cancer Institute, 1998c; Elmajian, 1997).

One of the reasons that Paclitaxel so intrigues cancer researchers is that it has an entirely new way of killing tumor cells. Paclitaxel works in a way that is exactly opposite to the vinca alkaloids: it prevents the microtubules from breaking back down into tubulin once their jobs are done (National Cancer Institute, 1998c; Medscape, 1997). A dividing cell forms the mitotic spindle, but is unable to break it down; this prevents the cell from finishing cell division. It becomes so crammed with unneeded microtubules that it simply stops functioning and dies (National Cancer Institute, 1998c). Figure 9.3 shows how this works. But Paclitaxel has other tricks up its sleeve, too. For example, cancer researchers have discovered that it is also a radiosensitizer for some (though not all) cancer cells in the laboratory (O'Shaughnessy, 1995; Aisner, 1997; Rosenthal, 1995). Clinical studies with Paclitaxel and radiotherapy are just beginning (Aisner, 1997). A newer relative of Paclitaxel has also been found. Docetaxel (Taxotene) manufactured from the needles of the European yew, *Taxus baccata*, appears to be even more effective than Paclitaxel (Anon, 1998b) and is being tested in clinical trials (Lavelle, 1995; National Cancer Institute, 1998c; Anon, 1998b).

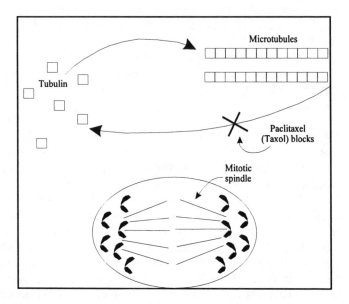

Figure 9.3. Paclitaxel blocks the breakdown of microtubules into tubulin, and stops cell division.

Paclitaxel is not a miracle cure for cancer, but it is very useful for some cancers with otherwise dismal cure rates. It first found a niche in the treatment of advanced (metastatic) breast cancers and ovarian cancers. These cancers respond as well (or better) to Paclitaxel alone as to standard treatments which combine several drugs (Medscape, 1997). From 20% - 62% of patients with metastatic breast cancer respond to Paclitaxel alone (0'shaughneassy, 1995; Stewart 1996). Up to 94 percent of breast cancer patients responded to a combination of Paclitaxel and Doxorubicin in a small preliminary study (Stewart, 1996). Ovarian cancer, particularly ovarian cancer which returns after treatment, has an extremely poor outlook; however, patients who are given Paclitaxel can gain months of extra time. In early cancer trials conducted at Johns Hopkins Medical center in 1989,some patients whose ovarian cancers returned after treatment gained an extra four to nine months with Paclitaxel (National Cancer Institute, 1998c). In a more recent study, 36 percent of patients responded to some extent to Paclitaxel, and 10 percent (3 of 33 patients) were still alive with no apparent disease, 12 months after Paclitaxel treatment (Nardi, 1996). Other studies of ovarian cancer have had similar success, with response rates from 20-37 percent (Nardi, 1996; Blom, 1996).

Paclitaxel and Docetaxel may also be effective against other types of cancer. They appear to have some activity against lung, head and neck, esophageal, bladder and colon cancers, as well as melanoma (Lavelle, 1995; Aisner, 1997; Rosenthal, 1995; National Cancer Institute, 1998c). Clinical trials are ongoing for many of the above cancers (National Cancer Institute, 1998c).

Thanks to such promising results, Paclitaxel has become a very popular drug. For a time, however, Paclitaxel use was crippled by a serious problem of availability. The Pacific yew is not abundant, does not grow particularly fast, and is found in protected old growth forests (Edwards, 1996). Furthermore, the concentration of Paclitaxel in the bark is very low (Edwards, 1996). Even if every yew were harvested, there is no way to grow yew trees fast enough to keep up with the demand for the bark.

Fortunately, there are now answers to this problem (Figure 9.4). Some researchers have found that a compound from the needles of the yew can be chemically altered to make Paclitaxel (Edwards, 1996). This new form of Paclitaxel is being tested in the clinics. Paclitaxel has also been synthesized completely from scratch (Edwards, 1996) although no companies seem to be using this technique yet. Finally, there may even be some hope from a lowly fungus. Researchers have found a fungus growing on yew trees, which seems to have picked up a gene from the tree and is capable of manufacturing Paclitaxel (Stierle, 1993). Fungi, unlike yew trees, can be grown abundantly and quickly in large batches in the laboratory.

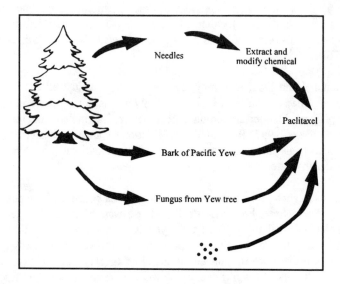

Figure 9.4. There are now a variety of ways to make Paclitaxel.

Although the supply problems seem to be solved, there remains much research to be done with Paclitaxel and Docetaxel. For example, researchers hope that combining Paclitaxel with other drugs might give even better responses than Paclitaxel alone (Medscape, 1997). There are currently phase I or II trials for Paclitaxel in combination with a number of drugs, including Cisplatin, 5-fluorouracil, and cyclophosphamide (Holmes, 1996) and Carboplatin (ten Bokkel, 1994). There have been promising early results combining Paclitaxel or Docetaxel with other drugs, but careful study is still needed to determine which combinations do work, and what side effects might develop with specific combinations (Aisner, 1997).

Related drugs from corals and bacteria -
eleutherobin and the epothilones

When Paclitaxel was first discovered, it seemed to be unique. Now, it seems that nature has been making a lot of different chemicals that can prevent microtubules from being broken back down into tubulin.

In an intriguing parallel to the Paclitaxel story, a new cancer cell killer has been found in a species of coral in the Indian Ocean (Anon, 1997). It is called eleutherobin and it works just like Paclitaxel. Although a drug company, Bristol-Myers Squibb, was interested enough in eleutherobin to obtain a license to manufacture the drug, there has been a problem. Corals, like yew trees, grow slowly. Just as the discovery of Paclitaxel threatened the yew tree with extinction, the discovery of eleutherobin has threatened these corals with extinction. Now, however, there is hope. K.C. Nicoleau and colleagues have managed to make eleutherobin from a chemical called carvone (Figure 9.5) - and carvone is obtained from the oil of dill or caraway seeds, far more abundant than corals (Anon, 1997).

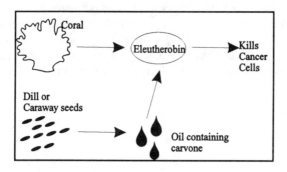

Figure 9.5. Eleutherobin, made from corals, or from dill or caraway seeds, can kill cancer cells.

Nicoleau's group has been busy. Recently, they made two more potential cancer killers from scratch (Nicoleau, 1997). These drugs, known as epothilones, were originally found in a bacterium, *Sorangium cellulosum*. They work like Paclitaxel, and prevent the microtubules from disassembling, but they may be effective even in cells which are resistant to Paclitaxel.

Interfering with proteins

Most of the drugs for cancer treatment interfere with DNA replication (or repair) or the manufacture of messenger RNA. A growing number interfere with microtubules. Finally, there are a few drugs which interfere with protein synthesis directly to poison the cancer cell. Asparaginase (Elspar), for example, is a drug which is particularly useful in leukemia. It destroys an amino acid (one of the building blocks necessary to make proteins) known as asparagine. Although all cells need asparagine, most can manufacture it; some cancer cells, however, cannot. Asparaginase destroys the asparagine in the blood, essentially starving the cancer cells. Another drug which interferes with proteins is homoharringtonine, a new drug made from the evergreen tree *Cephalotaxus harringtonin* (found in southern China) (Zhou, 1995). Homoharringtonine acts on the protein synthesis machinery (the ribosomes) to prevent them from making new proteins . In clinical studies, it has been effective for some leukemias.

Chapter 10

The problems with drugs - side effects and drug resistance

Traditional chemotherapy drugs walk a thin line: too little and they are ineffective, too much and they kill the patient. They are not subtle drugs. By interfering with processes found in all cells, they can kill any rapidly dividing cells. Fortunately, most of the time, cancer cells grow more quickly than normal cells; therefore, the normal cells tend to escape damage. However some normal cells do divide often and are, in fact, killed. These cells are often those which line the edges of the body. As a result, the cancer patient on chemotherapy may lose hair (the hair follicle cells die) with some drugs, or may develop a skin rash. Nausea and vomiting are common, and the mouth may become irritated and red, when cells lining the digestive tract are damaged.

The most dangerous side effect, however, is destruction of the cells in the bone marrow (Figure 10.1). When these cells are killed or damaged, fewer blood cells are made. If the red blood cell numbers fall too low, anemia results. If the numbers of platelets drops too far, the patient can bleed too easily. And if the white blood cells of the body diminish too much, infection can set in and could be deadly. Blood cell numbers are monitored during chemotherapy; dangerously low numbers signal the physician to stop or slow chemotherapy to allow the bone stem cells to recover. Sometimes, this can prevent a patient from receiving all of his or her chemotherapy.

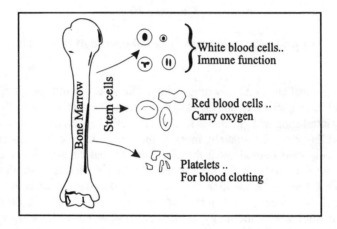

Figure 10.1. Stem cells in the bone marrow make all of the blood cells.

Other side effects are unique to particular drugs. Cyclophosphamide, one of the alkylating drugs, can occasionally cause bleeding in the urinary bladder. Cisplatin sometimes causes kidney problems and, once in a while, damage to hearing. The vinca alkaloids can interfere with nerve transmissions and cause difficulties with either sensation or control of muscles (Arioka, 1994). Paclitaxel also may occasionally cause problems with the nerves (National Cancer Institute, 1998c) The anthracylines such as Doxorubicin can cause heart damage. Researchers are currently testing newer relatives of many of these drugs, which have been designed to reduce these problems (Blomqvist, 1995; Arioka, 1994).

Treatment of side effects

Fortunately, scientists have found drugs which can counteract many of these side effects. These drugs can improve the quality of a patient's life during chemotherapy. They also allow chemotherapy drugs to be used longer and more effectively. Some new drugs (dexrazoxane/ICRF-187, amifostine/ Ethiofos, mesna, and ORG-2766) may be able to give patients some protection against some specific side effects (Lewis, 1994). Mesna, for example, may be able to protect the bladder against cyclophosphamide. A number of drugs can also control nausea and stop vomiting (Berkow,1992). These drugs might seem prosaic enough. But one potential new drug probably startled many people (Voth, 1997).

Crude marijuana, or a chemical found in marijuana, delta-9-tetrahydrocannabinol (THC) may be able to counteract nausea during chemotherapy and stimulate appetite in cancer patients (Voth, 1997). Some states have even considered legalizing marijuana for cancer patients. E.A. Voth and R.H. Schwartz. (1996) recently reviewed marijuana studies conducted between 1975 and 1996. Their conclusion is that these studies support the investigation of THC, at least, to treat nausea and stimulate appetite; they don't, however, support the reclassification of marijuana itself as a prescription drug.

While some side effects make a patient miserable, bone marrow destruction is potentially deadly. At one time, the only solution, other than stopping the drugs and allowing the bone marrow to recover on its own, was a blood transfusion. Although blood transfusions can replace red blood cells and platelets, they are not very effective at replacing white blood cells: immune cells simply don't work well in someone else's body (Glaspy, 1997; Berkow, 1992). Transfusions also carry the risk of potentially deadly allergic reactions to someone else's blood (called transfusion reactions) and a slight risk of infection by some viruses. Recent developments have, however, reduced the need for transfusions and also given physicians a way to boost white blood cell levels.

These "wonder drugs" are cytokines, proteins made by the immune system. Some of these cytokines instruct the bone marrow to make blood cells; they can be used to treat patients whose blood cell levels drop too low. Erythropoietin (Epoetin alpha), for example, can boost red blood cell levels (Glaspy, 1997). In some recent studies, Erythropoietin decreased the need for transfusions in some patients treated with chemotherapy, and improved their energy (Glaspy, 1997). Two other cytokines, G-CSF (granulocyte colony stimulating factor) and GM-CSF (granulocyte monocyte colony stimulating factor) have been used to prevent infections. Although G-CSF and GM-CSF have slightly different effects on the white cell population, they both increase the numbers of a major bacteria-fighting cell, the neutrophil. These cytokines have been able to decrease both the number of infections and the length of hospitalization after chemotherapy (Ezaki, 1997). Recently, several studies have shown that another cytokine, called interleukin 6, may be able to prevent or decrease the drop in platelet numbers during chemotherapy (Schuler, 1996; D'Hondt, 1995).

Melatonin, a hormone from the pineal gland, may also be useful for the treatment of bone marrow suppression. In a pilot study, melatonin was given to patients with various types of metastatic tumors who were in poor health (Lissoni, 1997). Forty patients were treated with the standard chemotherapy for their particular type of cancer, and the other forty received the same chemotherapy with the addition of melatonin. The patients given melatonin had fewer episodes of low platelet counts, and generally felt better. Unfortunately, melatonin did not affect other side effects such as hair loss and vomiting.

Cancer treatments that cause cancer?

Finally, there is a potentially serious problem which happens not at the time of treatment, but perhaps many years in the future. It lies in the fact that many of the cytotoxic drugs damage DNA. As you may recall, the root cause of cancer is a mutation in a critical gene; in other words, DNA damage. Why don't the cytotoxic drugs cause new cancers to form? In fact, once in a while, they may. Cyclophosphamide, for instance, has been linked to bladder cancers (Boffetta, 1994). The DNA alkylating drugs may also increase the chance of lymphomas and lung cancer (Boffetta, 1994; Salmon, 1987). Unfortunately, these drugs are among the most effective anti-cancer drugs. So, at this time, it may be worth the risk of possible cancer in the future, in return for the cure of a cancer which will certainly kill now.

Drug resistance

There is another serious problem with chemotherapy drugs. This problem is that, sometimes, the cancer cells stop being affected by the drug (Figure 10.2). This phenomenon is known as drug resistance. Some cancer cells seem to come with drug resistance before they're ever exposed to the drug; melanoma, kidney cancers, cancers of the pancreas, and some brain tumors are notorious for this (Berkow, 1992; Patel, 1994). Other cancers may develop resistance after treatment with drugs. Sometimes, drug resistance develops only to a single drug, and switching drugs may work. Too often, however, treatment with one drug is followed by the development of drug resistance not only to that drug, but also to a number of other drugs. This is known as multiple drug resistance and is depressingly common. One report estimates that drug resistance is the single most common reason for treatment failure during cancer therapy (Patel, 1994).

Resistance to a single drug

Resistance to a single drug often occurs when the target of that drug either mutates or increases in amount in the cell. For example, cancer cells can become resistant to the vinca alkaloids when their microtubules mutate. The altered microtubules are no longer affected by the vinca alkaloids, and the cell now simply ignores the drug. In other cases, the target does not change, but there is much more of it in a cell, enough to overcome the actions of the drug. It is as if ten molecules of drug, which were previously fighting ten molecules of target, now have to contend with thousands of targets. They simply can't keep up. Usually, this happens when the cell makes many extra copies of the target gene in a cell, although occasionally a single gene can also become overactive (el-Deiry, 1997).

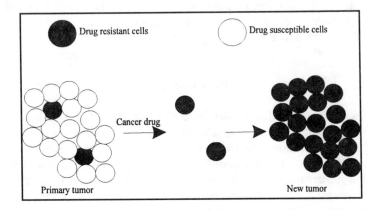

Figure 10.2. Although drugs can kill many of the cells in a tumor, drug resistant cells can remain behind and form a new, more resistant tumor.

Resistance to multiple drugs

Multiple drug resistance is a more serious problem than single drug resistance, because now several whole groups of drugs may have become ineffective against the cancer cell. This group may include drugs with very different activities and chemical structures. For example, resistance can develop simultaneously to the anthracyclines (Doxorubicin and its relatives), vinca alkaloids, and a group of drugs called the epipodophyllotoxins (Etoposide and Eniposide) (Nooter, 1996). Often, after multiple drug resistance develops, the options for effective drugs shrink dramatically. In fact, for some cancers, there may be no effective drugs left. Researchers are hoping to learn how multiple drug resistance works, in order to prevent or to defeat it. One clue is the recent finding that there is more than one way to develop multiple drug resistance (Nooter, 1996).

In one common type of multiple drug resistance, cancer cells make proteins to pump out drug molecules as soon as they enter the cell (Cress, 1996; Nooter, 1996; Fisher, 1995; el-Deiry, 1997). They expel the drugs before they even have a chance to work (Figure 10.3). The pumps, called Pgp proteins, can work on many different drugs; therefore, when the number of Pgp proteins in a cell increases, resistance to many different drugs can develop simultaneously. A different protein, from the *mrp* gene, also seems to be involved in resistance, although little is known about how it works (Nooter, 1996; el-Deiry, 1997). Some researchers think that the Mrp protein works like Pgp and removes drugs from the cell, or possibly locks them away into some compartment of the cell where they can do no harm (Nooter, 1996; el-Deiry, 1997). There are also other ways that multiple drug resistance develops. For example, the cancer cell can increase its ability to destroy cancer drugs that have entered the cell (el-Deiry, 1997). Cancer cells can also develop resistance to some drugs by increasing their DNA repair enzymes and simply correcting any damage that occurs (Grosland, 1996; el-Deiry, 1997).

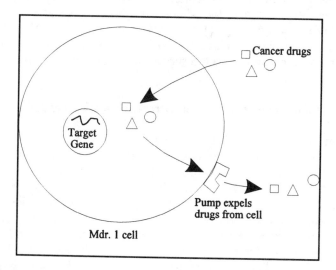

Figure 10.3. The Pgp pump can expel cancer drugs from the cell before they do any damage.

Fighting back against drug resistance

Cancer researchers are very interested in finding ways to reverse multiple drug resistance. Clinical trials of drugs to reverse multiple drug resistance due to the Pgp protein have begun. Unfortunately, so far, the drugs have not been completely successful (Fisher, 1995). There have, however, been some encouraging results in cancers of the blood (Fisher, 1995). One of the more promising drugs, SDZ PSC 833, is in numerous phase I and II clinical trials, in combination with a variety of drugs, including Paclitaxel. Gene therapy to turn off the gene for Pgp (called the *mdr-1* gene) is also a goal of investigators (Davis, 1996).

Researchers are also struggling to find ways to reverse other forms of resistance. For example, drugs have been given to inhibit DNA repair, or the cell's ability to destroy drugs (Grosland, 1996). A phase II trial to determine whether resistance to the DNA alkylating drugs can be overcome has met with very limited success (Tetef, 1995). In this study, patients with drug resistant tumors were given a DNA alkylating drug. Patients were also given Menadione, a drug which suppresses the cell's ability to detoxify drugs (Tetef, 1995). Only two of the 23 patients responded to this combination (two others may have had very brief responses), and average patient survival was not significantly improved.

Using drug resistance to increase chemotherapy doses

Some researchers would like to exploit drug resistance genes from cancer cells. They want to use them to make normal cells resistant to the side effects of chemotherapy. One gene that has been suggested is the gene for the PGP pump, the *mdr-1* gene (Davis, 1996). Researchers hope to put the *mdr-1* gene into enough normal cells to repopulate an organ quickly if the normal, unmodified cells die. In fact, the *mdr-1* gene has successfully been put into bone marrow cells in a variety of experiments (Davis, 1996). It seems to be able to keep bone marrow alive in mice treated with chemotherapy drugs: in one experiment, mice without the *mdr-1* gene in their stem cells had a 93 percent drop in bone marrow stem cells after chemotherapy, but mice with the gene showed no drop at all (Davis, 1996).

Getting away from the cytotoxic drugs -
the new drug arsenal against cancer

At the moment, the cytotoxic drugs are often the most effective drugs available to treat many cancers. Yet, as we have seen, they have many problems. They tend to be extremely toxic. They have problems with drug resistance. And they are not always effective. Some people wonder whether, someday, our descendants will look back on our current treatment of cancer much as we look back on the use of leeches. "They used drugs related to chemical warfare weapons?!" they will ask in disbelief. In the remainder of the book, we will be looking at an incredible variety of new drugs. There are drugs which block cancer cells from migrating, drugs which attack the tumor blood vessels and drugs which stimulate the immune system. There are drugs which use light to destroy cancer cells. There is even a technique called hyperthermia, where a simple fever can shrink tumors. Some of the newest cancer treatments may not, however, depend on new drugs. They may simply be ways of using the old drugs in new and unusual ways. In the next few chapters, we will look at new ways of delivering drugs to tumors, how the time of day may affect drug safety and effectiveness, and how giving life-threatening doses of drugs can cure some cancers.

Building the highways instead of the cars -
changing how drugs are given

Cancer researchers have noticed a problem. Sometimes, drugs which look very promising in preclinical trials don't live up to that promise in the human cancer patients (Jain, 1996). One reason is that mice and humans are different creatures, with slightly different body functions. These slight differences can affect where drugs are delivered in the body, and how and when they are removed from the body. Some researchers suspect that some drugs which worked in mice do not reach human cancers in effective quantities. Rakesh K Jain (1996) likens it to cars on a highway. We could have the most sophisticated, elaborate cars in the world; but without roads that allow those cars to reach their destinations, they would be utterly useless. Some current drug research focuses on delivering the drugs more effectively and safely to the tumor, rather than on making new drugs to use. In other words, building the highways, instead of the cars.

Drug delivery to tumors

The amount of drug actually reaching cancer cells depends on many factors. It can be helpful to think of it as two antagonistic systems working on the drug: one to deliver the drug to the tumor, and the other to remove it from the body.

Drug delivery to cancer cells is a complicated process. Most drugs are delivered to tumors by the bloodstream. If the drug is taken by mouth or injected under the skin, only a portion of the drug will make it into the blood. Even a drug injected directly into the blood (as most cancer drugs are), is not delivered equally to all of the cells in the body. Blood flow varies between areas of the body, as does the ability of drugs to escape from the blood into the fluids surrounding cells. It can be particularly difficult to get some drugs to the cells of a tumor (Hall, 1995). Tumor blood vessels can behave very oddly (Hall, 1995). For example, in normal organs, the pressure inside the blood vessel is higher than outside, helping to force fluids (and the important molecules they carry) from the blood vessel to the surrounding cells. In tumors, however, the pressure in the tumor can be as high as in the blood vessel. This can make it difficult for large molecules inside the blood vessel to get outside to the tumor cells.

The second set of forces acting on the drug are the body systems which remove foreign substances from the body. The two organs which clear most substances from the body are the liver and the kidneys. The liver detoxifies some drugs. It modifies other drugs into forms that can be more easily removed from the blood, and removes some drugs directly, by sending them to the intestine. The kidneys filter the blood, removing drugs and other substances into the urine.

The net result of these two sets of forces is that, at any given time, some of the drug is being delivered to the tumor, while some of the drug is being removed from body. An equilibrium exists between the amount of drug in the tumor, the blood, and other sites. The amount of drug being delivered to the tumor will gradually increase, then decrease as the kidneys and/or liver remove and detoxify the drug. Eventually, all of the drug will leave the body.

Why different people react differently to a drug

As we all know, people can vary quite a bit. While this variability makes our lives more interesting, it also causes a headache for physicians who treat cancer. Although most chemotherapy is given at a standard dose (adjusting for body size and for any co-existing diseases), people do not react identically to that dose (van Warmerdam, 1997; Masson, 1997). With a standard dose, the amount of drug being delivered to the tumor can easily vary between any two people (van Warmerdam, 1997).There are a number of reasons for this. For example, the drug must be able to get from the blood to the cancer; this depends on blood flow to the particular tumor, the state of the patient's circulatory system in general, and other factors.

Recently, there has been interest in adjusting drug doses for each individual patient. By doing so, researchers hope to minimize side effects and ensure that equal amounts of drug actually reach the tumor in all patients.

Unfortunately, it would be impossible to calculate all of factors which affect drug delivery, for each dose. Half a dozen different enzymes in the liver, for example, may act on a single drug - and that's not even considering kidney function, which can even vary depending on the time of day! A simple way to individualize drugs, however, is to adjust the dose to maintain steady levels of the drug in an individual's blood (van Warmerdam, 1997). Although this technique does not guarantee that drug is actually reaching all of the cells of the tumor, it does eliminate some of the variability. Several drugs, including Methotrexate and Carboplatin, can currently be individualized for each patient (Masson, 1997). Others such as 5-fluorouracil, Etoposide, and Topotecan may eventually be individualized as well (Masson, 1997).

Giving drugs directly into the tumor

Drugs given into the bloodstream, as we have seen, are not always delivered well to tumors. Although individualizing drug doses may help, some researchers would like to bypass the whole complicated mess and just give the drug directly into the tumor. One technique is to inject the drug into the blood vessels supplying the organ where the tumor is found. This can decrease some of the variability in drug dosing, and it can also reduce the side effects. In one study from China, 14 patients with various cancers of the reproductive tract were given their drug doses directly into the blood vessels supplying the reproductive organs (Zhao, 1994). These patients were able to receive a higher dose of the drugs with fewer side effects; their cancers also responded better than to conventional chemotherapy. A twist on this approach is to enclose the cancer drugs inside tiny capsules (just as many over the counter drugs are packaged in capsules), and place the capsules into the blood vessels feeding the tumors. In this way, researchers have been able to target tumors in the liver, kidney, head and neck, bone, and internal organs in the pelvis (Kato, 1996). This technique is still very new, but in one group of 427 patients, it seemed to be promising (Kato, 1996). A few people (0.9%) had serious complications from treatment (including two ˙ deaths); however, considering the serious condition of most of the patients, the treatment was fairly successful. The treatments reduced symptoms and improved the quality of life for two thirds of the patients given mitomycin C. In 28 percent of the participants, the tumors shrunk by at least half. The authors suggest clinical trials to further evaluate this therapy.

Another approach is to give drugs in carriers which can be implanted at the tumor site and will slowly release the drug to the tumor. Plachitin is a combination of the cancer drug Cisplatin and a substance in insect and crab skeletons known as chitin (Suzuki, 1995). When Plachitin was implanted into tumors in mice, it produced a high concentration of Cisplatin in the surrounding tumor tissues, but without the kidney damage that would be expected if such high doses had resulted from conventional treatment (Suzuki, 1995). Survival was also improved.

Chapter 11

Magic Bullets -
targeting tumor cells with antibodies and other carriers

There is, however, an even more intriguing way to get drugs to cancer cells than to use crab skeletons: have them delivered by antibodies.

What is an antibody?

Antibodies are proteins made by white blood cells called B lymphocytes. As immunologists are fond of telling their students, an antibody looks roughly like the letter "Y". The two arms on top of the antibody can each grasp and hold another molecule; in natural antibodies, the two arms always attach to exactly the same molecule. The molecules which antibodies grab are called, for convenience, antigens. Each antibody molecule can only attach to one antigen and to no others (Figure 11.1). For example, an antibody which grabs a protein on the *Salmonella* bacterium cannot attach to a different antigen on the bacterium which causes cholera.

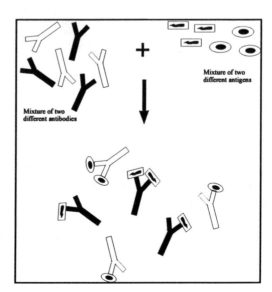

Figure 11.1. Each antibody can attach to only one antigen.

Magic bullets

The natural function of an antibody is to fight infections; however, a long time ago, researchers realized the potential for antibodies to deliver chemicals to specific cells. If, they reasoned, a chemical poison or drug could be attached to the right antibody (Figure 11.2), then the antibody would carry the chemical directly to the cancer cells - and only to the cancer cells. Antibodies have been used to carry drugs, radioactive atoms, and a variety of toxins (cell poisons) in experimental cancer therapy. These hybrid molecules are often called immunotoxins - or, sometimes, magic bullets.

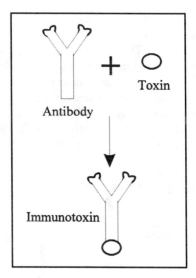

Figure 11.2.

Good immunotoxins are difficult to make, but very simple to use. They are usually just injected into the bloodstream. If the antibody has been chosen well, the immunotoxins should all end up at the site of the cancer cells, carrying their lethal burdens. In this way, most of the drug or toxin or radioactivity can be concentrated on the cancer cells, with very little exposure to normal cells. Side effects should be minimized, and much higher doses seen at the actual cancer site.

Immunotoxins have been tested in laboratory animals and also used in clinical cancers for more than 20 years (Frankel, 1995). Unfortunately, although some results using immunotoxins in mice have been impressive, most human trials have not been spectacular (Pietersz, 1994). Several recent reviews sum up the overall situation as "encouraging, but needs more work" (Frankel, 1995; Pietersz, 1994 Uckun, 1995). There have, however, been some isolated successes. Immunotoxins may be particularly useful for cancers of the blood, where cells are more accessible than in solid tumor masses (Uckun, 1995; Frankel, 1995). Recently, an antibody carrying a radioactive iodine molecule (I^{131}) was dramatically successful in patients with one type of leukemia (Hall, 1995). In the first tests with this antibody, all evidence of cancer disappeared in 16 of 19 patients. Eight patients were still free of cancer three and a half to eight years later, and may be cured. In a second trial with this antibody, 17 of 21 patients went into complete remission. Unfortunately, the large dose of antibody that was needed for such good results also killed normal immune cells; bone marrow transplants were needed to save the patients after treatment.

A new refinement has now allowed researchers to give lower doses of antibody, while maintaining the effectiveness of the therapy (Hall, 1995). Researchers knew that some organs, such as the liver and spleen, absorbed large amounts of the antibodies injected into the blood. In the first experiments, extra antibodies had to be given to fill up these "sinks," in addition to the dose needed to reach the cancer cells. In the new experiments, patients were first given the antibodies, but with no I^{131} attached. These antibodies filled up all of the places where the immunotoxins usually go, such as the spleen and liver, before they reach the tumor tissue. The patients were then given low doses of an antibody with I^{131} - which promptly bypassed all other sites and homed in on the cancer cells. Twenty two of 28 patients responded to this treatment. Fourteen of them were complete responses, many of which have lasted more than a year. The bone marrow was suppressed, but recovered without transplants. And the patients went home in three days, instead of a month.

Problems, pitfalls, and solutions

Most of the problems with immunotoxins have resulted from an unfortunate tendency for them to find their way to places besides the cancer. The toxins have damaged normal tissues and resulted in leaky blood vessels, liver damage and nervous system damage (Frankel, 1995).

Another problem is that immunotoxins are rather bulky molecules and sometimes have difficulty getting inside tumors (Frankel, 1995). A final problem is that the patient's immune system sometimes reacts to the immunotoxins (much as it would to anything not normally found in the body) and eliminates them before they can do any good (Frankel, 1995). Researchers are developing better immunotoxins to overcome these problems. In some cases, this means making smaller immunotoxins which can more easily penetrate inside the tumor. In other cases, antibodies are being refined to attach more tightly to cancer cells. Finally, new "humanized" antibodies make it less likely that the immune system itself will prevent the immunotoxin from doing its job.

Single chain toxins - slimming antibodies down

One way to make immunotoxins a bit less bulky, and perhaps more effective, is to engineer an antibody molecule called a single chain antibody, which has only one attachment site for antigen. This slimmed down molecule can more easily slip into the centers of tumors. Some single chain immunotoxins are being tested in preclinical trials. A single chain antibody which attaches to an oncogene called HER-2 has been able to destroy breast cancer cells in the laboratory and cause tumor regression in laboratory animal models (King, 1996). Other single chain immunotoxins or small antibody fragments have been effective either against cells in the laboratory (Kreitman, 1994) or against tumors in mice (Kuan, 1996).

Half mouse/ half human antibodies

One significant problem with antibodies used in cancer treatment is that they are made by mouse cells. The human immune system sees these mouse antibodies and recognizes that they do not belong inside the human body; it, therefore, eliminates them. This phenomenon can limit treatment with antibodies to a single treatment (Hall, 1995). The second time around, the immune response can eliminate them too quickly for them to do any good. It can also cause some nasty side effects, depending on the dose: joint aches, fever, damaged blood vessels and even kidney problems. The solution to this problem seems to be the development of "humanized" antibodies.

Humanized antibodies (Figure 11.3) are a hybrid of mouse and human antibodies (Hall,1995; Kuby, 1997). An antibody molecule is made up of the two ends which attach to the antigen, and the rest of the molecule, which serves as more or less a framework for the antigen attachment sites. With genetic engineering, a mouse B cell can be used to make the antigen attachment sites, but the framework can be mostly replaced with the framework for a human antibody . Since most of the molecule is now of human origin, the human immune system is much less likely to react to it.

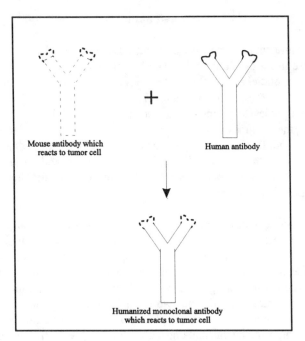

Figure 11.3. Humanized monoclonal antibodies can be made by combining mouse and human antibodies.

Non-antibody molecules which deliver toxins

In some cases, molecules other than antibodies can be used to guide a toxin to cancer cells (although it may be more difficult to find molecules which do not also attach to normal cells). For example, a toxin linked to the protein IL-2 has been used to treat lymphocyte cancers which did not respond to conventional therapy (Tepler, 1994). IL-2 is a normal product of the immune system. It attaches only to lymphocytes which are actively dividing. Researchers, therefore, expected the toxin to be guided to the cancerous lymphocytes or to other actively dividing lymphocytes, but not to other "resting" lymphocytes. In this Phase I/II study, the guided toxin appeared to be partially successful. One patient out of 15 had a complete response to therapy lasting more than two years. Many other types of guidance molecules are also being tried.

Prodrugs

Researchers are also developing other new techniques to make sure that cancer drugs kill cancer cells but ignore normal cells. One promising new method is to inject "prodrugs," nontoxic chemicals which can be converted into toxic drugs by specific enzymes. Prodrugs are harmless to a cell, unless it contains the enzyme which converts it to the toxic form. The trick, therefore, is to make a prodrug which will be converted by enzymes found in cancer cells, but not in normal cells (as shown in figure 11.4.)

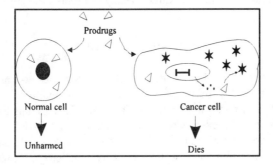

Figure 11.4. Inside cancer cells, prodrugs are converted into active drugs and kill the cell.

One approach is to look for naturally occurring enzymes in tumors and select drugs which are converted by them. For example, one enzyme found in many tumors is β-glucuronidase (Murdter, 1997). A prodrug called HMR1826 can be converted by β-glucuronidase into the cancer drug Doxorubicin (Murdter, 1997). Theoretically, if HMR1826 was given to a patient with a β-glucuronidase-containing tumor, the tumor cells should convert HMR1826 into toxic Doxorubicin, but normal cells would see only the nontoxic unmodified drug. In this way, the side effects of Doxorubicin treatment, notably damage to the heart, could be avoided and higher, more effective doses could be given. HMR1826 is still very new and has not yet been tested in the clinics. It was, however, promising in a model of the human lung (Murdter, 1997). In this model, normal cells usually absorb more Doxorubicin than tumor cells; however, when HMR1826 was injected instead, cancers accumulated seven times as much Doxorubicin as the normal cells around the tumor.

In general, however, it is quite difficult to find a useful enzyme, present only in tumors, which will convert prodrugs into toxic drugs. So, sometimes, researchers find a way to get the enzyme into the tumor cell artificially. One way is to carry the enzyme to the tumor cells with an approach known as antibody-directed enzyme prodrug therapy (ADEPT).

ADEPT and ADAPT

ADEPT uses antibodies to deliver chosen enzymes to cancer cells (Wentworth, 1996). In a way, it's a twist on immunotoxins; however, instead of carrying the toxin itself, the antibody delivers only the enzyme to make a prodrug toxic. A recent variation, called ADAPT, does away with the enzyme molecule, for fear that it could stimulate an immune response which eliminates it. Instead, it uses an "abzyme", an unusual antibody which itself acts as an enzyme. Abzyme antibodies are not naturally found in the body, but are manufactured in the laboratory. ADAPT treatment is very new, but it has been able to kill human colon cancer cells in the laboratory (Wentworth, 1996).

Chapter 12

Circadian rhythms -
how our internal clocks affect cancer drugs

One of the most amazing discoveries in biology is that our bodies have an internal clock. Blood flow, hormone secretion and many other activities increase and decrease daily in a roughly 24 hour cycle (Focan, 1995; Bjarnason, 1995). This 24 hour cycle is called a circadian rhythm and it seems to be a part of every cell (Focan, 1995; Bjarnason, 1995). Patterns of light and dark reset the cycle every day, but even in continual darkness, it persists (Bjarnason, 1995). It is genetically controlled; mutating certain genes can change the length of the cycle or its sensitivity to light (Bjarnason, 1995). We share it with all other living things, from the smallest amoeba to the tallest redwood tree (Bjarnason, 1995). It may even be an important part of cancer treatment someday.

Quite a bit of evidence suggests that some cancer drugs may be most effective and least toxic when they are given at certain times of the day (Focan, 1995; Bjarnason, 1995). The explanation for this phenomenon lies in the circadian rhythms of the cells. From animal experiments as well as studies on humans, biologists have found that cells in each organ divide in a rhythmic pattern. At some times of the day, many cells are dividing; at others, most are quiet (Focan, 1995; Bjarnason, 1995). Each organ seems to have its own pattern. For example, in humans, most cell division in the bone marrow occurs between the hours of 7 am and 4 pm, while, in the intestines, the peak activity seems to be between 5 and 9 am (Bjarnason, 1995). Tumors, too seem to have circadian rhythms (although they may lose them as the cancer advances); cell division in early tumors seems to occur in waves of activity and inactivity scheduled at specific times of the day (Focan, 1995).

If you recall, most chemotherapy drugs specifically destroy dividing cells, not resting cells. The idea behind circadian therapy is to give the drug at a time when many cancer cells are dividing, but few normal cells are. In this way, the ability of the drug to kill cancer cells can be maximized, while the side effects are minimized. One complicating factor is, however, that body processes besides cell division have circadian rhythms. The activity of the liver and kidneys, which eliminate many cancer drugs, varies with the time of day (Focan, 1995; Bjarnason, 1995). Blood flow to tumors may also change over time: in rats (which are active at night), tumor blood flow can be twice as high at night as during the day (Bjarnason, 1995). Even the ability of normal cells to detoxify the drug may vary (Bjarnazson, 1995). Many other processes that affect drug levels also change during the day (Bjarnason, 1995). Ultimately, the best time for a drug dose depends not only on cell division patterns, but on all of the factors that affect drug delivery and elimination from the body. For this reason, determining the optimal time for drug doses can be a complicated process.

Most circadian therapy experiments have, to this point, been done in laboratory animals such as rats and mice. In these animals, the time of least toxicity (fewest side effects) has been determined for many chemotherapy agents (Focan, 1995). In some cases, the ability of the drug to kill cancer cells is also better when it is given at certain times of the day. For example, in one experiment, Cisplatin produced complete regressions in 60 percent of tumors in laboratory rodents when it was given at the optimal time, but only in 20 percent when it was given at another time (Focan, 1995). Not all chemotherapy drugs vary in toxicity or effectiveness with time (Focan, 1995; Bjarnason, 1995); however, many common drugs, including Paclitaxel, 5-fluorouracil, Doxorubicin, Vincristine, and many others, seem to be good candidates for circadian therapy.

Circadian therapy is slowly moving into clinical trials in humans. This process does, however, have its stumbling blocks. One problem is that humans and laboratory animals are active during opposite times of the day: mice and rats, unlike humans, are nocturnal. Sometimes, researchers try to give drugs to humans 12 hours later than in mice (Focan, 1995).

This may, however, be no better than a first guess and the best time in humans must still be determined experimentally. Another problem is that individual humans seem to be considerably more variable than mice; optimal times often vary between individuals (Focan, 1995). Finally, sometimes humans seem to lose some of their circadian rhythms as the cancer progresses. Not only may the tumor lose its cyclic pattern of cell division, but even normal blood cell production may no longer occur in a regular pattern (Focan, 1995).

Nevertheless, circadian therapy in humans has shown promise, particularly in early cancers. In one study, children with one type of leukemia (acute lymphocytic leukemia) were allowed to take their maintenance drugs in either the evening or the morning: those who took their drugs in the evening had a better response (Focan, 1995). In other studies, patients with metastatic kidney cancer or colon cancer were given their drugs either at steady doses over several hours, or at a dose which varied and was highest at the optimum circadian time (Bjarnason, 1995). The drugs were less toxic when they were administered at the variable dose than when they were given at the steady rate. In the colon cancer study, 50 percent of the patients who received the variable rate also had at least a partial response to treatment, while only 30 percent responded to the steady rate. Several other studies have also shown that some drugs have fewer side effects in humans when they are given at particular times of the day or night (Focan, 1995; Bjarnason, 1995). Further clinical trials are in progress (Focan, 1995; Bjarnason, 1995).

Circadian therapy is still in its infancy. Before it can become routine, a number of problems remain to be worked out. Too little is known yet about human circadian rhythms, and the optimal times of drug dosing. Individual variability must also somehow be predicted and considered in treatment plans. The loss in circadian rhythms in advanced cancers is a significant problem; circadian therapy may turn out to be ineffective where it is needed most. One final practical consideration is that circadian rhythms do not respect normal business hours. Sometimes, the optimal time for a drug may be in the middle of the night, when few doctors are in their practices and, even in hospitals, fewer personnel are available.

Yet, in spite of problems to be solved, and additional research to be done, circadian therapy is an intriguing idea. It's a wonderful thought that, perhaps a simple matter of changing the timing of a medication could diminish the side effects and increase the chance of beating the cancer.

Chapter 13

Giving life-threatening doses of drugs - high dose chemotherapy

All chemotherapy drugs have side effects which limit the dose that can be given. If the doses are too high, the patient dies of the treatment instead of the disease. For many chemotherapy drugs, the side effect limiting the dose is the destruction of the patient's bone marrow. Without enough red blood cells to carry oxygen, white blood cells to fight infection, or platelets to start blood clotting, a person will surely die. The cells that produce white blood cells, red blood cells, and platelets are found in the bone marrow; as a group, they are called stem cells. Under normal conditions, stem cells are constantly dividing and renewing the body's supply of blood cells. Because of this, they are exquisitely sensitive to drugs which damage DNA or stop cell division. Low doses of chemotherapy drugs kill some of these cells; high doses can kill all of them. Often, chemotherapy must be stopped or delayed because the blood cells have dropped to dangerously low levels.

With some types of cancer, the chances of a cure with such "safe" doses of chemotherapy are very slim. The conventional dose may not be enough to kill all of the cancer cells - but any higher dose would kill the patient more surely than the cancer will. This is a dilemma that has troubled physicians and cancer researchers for some time. Now a drastic solution offers hope to some patients.

This solution is a new approach to chemotherapy called "high dose chemotherapy with stem cell support" (Vaughan, 1997; Stewart, 1996). In this form of chemotherapy, very high doses of drugs are given: doses which, researchers hope, will kill all of the cancer cells in the body. Such doses will also kill all of the stem cells in the bone marrow. Therefore, before the drugs are given, the patient donates a bone marrow sample; these cells are safely preserved outside the body until after the drugs have been given (Figure 13.1). Sometimes, a blood sample is taken instead, since stem cells are also found in the blood (Stewart, 1996; Vaughan, 1997). After the amount of the drug in the body has fallen to safe levels, the stem cells are returned to the body. The gamble is that the drug will eliminate all of the tumor cells, and that the stem cells will successfully return to the bone marrow and start producing blood cells before a deadly infection can set in.

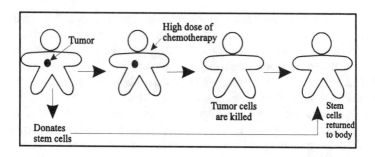

Figure 13.1. High dose chemotherapy: before treatment with high doses of drugs, the patient donates stem cells, which are returned at the end of therapy.

This procedure might like seem a desperate solution. But the risks are balanced by a chance of a cure in patients who otherwise have little or no hope. It seems to work, sometimes, in some lymphomas and a brain tumor known as neuroblastoma (National Cancer Institute, 1998c). It also shows promise in high risk breast cancers (Stewart, 1996; Vaughan, 1997) and ovarian cancers (Stewart, 1996; Vaughan, 1997).

The results in advanced breast cancer

High dose chemotherapy has been mainly used for cancers where the chances of survival or cure are otherwise slim. One such cancer is advanced breast cancer, where metastasis has spread the tumor far beyond the breast. Traditional chemotherapy for advanced breast cancer can completely suppress only 5 to 25% of tumors (Stewart, 1996). Most of these cancers will eventually return; the average remission is only 5 to 13 months. Stem cell transplants, however, allow the doses of chemotherapy drugs to be increased to five to ten times the normal dose, and these higher doses appear to be killing breast cancer cells more effectively (Stewart, 1996).

In the largest clinical trials, tumors disappeared in thirty five to 68% of patients with metastatic breast cancer (Stewart, 1996). Unfortunately, the cancer returned in 6 to 12 months in most patients, just as it returns with conventional treatment. A minority of the patients, however, were more fortunate; 19% to 27% of the group survived for 4 years. A few were still alive, with no sign of disease, more than five years later. In fact, in one group of 22 patients, three patients were alive and healthy nine to twelve years after they had been treated. Such statistics might not seem such a good odds; but, when you consider the poor outlook with conventional chemotherapy, many of us might choose to gamble that we would fall into that lucky few percent.

Recently, several clinical trials to compare high dose chemotherapy to conventional chemotherapy have begun (Stewart, 1996). Results are available from one of these trials (Stewart, 1996). In this trial, 90 patients with metastatic breast cancer were treated with either standard chemotherapy or with high dose chemotherapy with stem cell support. Although more patients in this trial responded to the high dose treatment than to conventional chemotherapy, most of them soon progressed again in spite of treatment. But, just as in the earlier studies, a small number of patients survived for years and may have been cured with the high dose treatment; no patients were cured with the conventional treatment. The results are summarized in the table below.

* *

Table 13.1

	High Dose Chemotherapy	Standard Chemotherapy
Overall response rate	93%	53%
Complete response rate	51%	4%
Median survival	90 weeks	45 weeks
3 year survival without recurrence of disease	17%	0%

The overall response rate is the percentage of patients whose tumors shrunk with treatment (whether partially or completely); the complete response rate is the percentage of patients whose tumors completely disappeared, at least for a while. Median survival is one type of measurement of average survival (defined more fully in the glossary).

* *

Some researchers suspect that high dose chemotherapy may work even better in patients whose cancer is in earlier stages. One group of researchers treated women with locally advanced breast cancer; these were women who had signs of cancer in their lymph nodes but no obvious metastasis elsewhere (Stewart, 1996). Of these women, 31 to 34 % would have been expected to survive for five years without further signs of breast cancer with conventional treatment. With high dose chemotherapy, 71% did. A new study tested high dose chemotherapy in women with even fewer metastasis in their lymph nodes (four to nine metastasis in comparison to 10 or more in the previous study); 80-90% of these women were still alive two to three years later, with no signs of disease (Stewart, 1996).

The results in ovarian cancer

High dose chemotherapy is also being tried in patients with ovarian cancer, another cancer where the outlook for long term survival can be poor. Fewer than 20 women out of every 100 with metastatic ovarian cancer survive for 5 years (Stewart, 1996). Although the cancer may go into remission, it often returns. Those patients who relapse have little hope; although 20 to 30% will respond to treatment, less than 5% will be alive without evidence of cancer progression 2 years later (Stewart, 1996). Some researchers, however, believe that high dose chemotherapy may be an option for such patients. Although there have been few published reports on high dose chemotherapy in ovarian cancer patients, one small study was promising. In 30 patients treated with high dose chemotherapy, 89% responded at least partially, and seven of the 30 were still alive with no signs of disease three years later (Stewart, 1996). In other studies, four of 18 patients, and two of five patients, were alive without apparent tumors six to 12 months later (Stewart, 1996). High dose chemotherapy has also been tried as the initial treatment for ovarian cancer. In one very encouraging study, 57% of patients with advanced ovarian cancer were still alive without signs of disease 4 years later (Stewart, 1996).

The risks

High dose chemotherapy is not without risks. High doses of drugs can also have unexpected and very toxic side effects on organs other than the bone marrow. There is also a chance that the patient will die from an overwhelming infection before the returned stem cells find their way back to the bone marrow and successfully colonize it. Between 1992 and 1994, approximately four out of every 100 patients who received their own bone marrow died within 100 days after the transplant (thanks to better supportive care and other advances, this rate has dropped dramatically since 1989 to 1991, when sixteen out of every 100 died) (Stewart, 1996). Even those who do not have major side effects from the transplant, however, will undergo considerable discomfort and expense.

Another major concern is that cancer cells may be hiding among the stem cells. Sometimes, cancer cells can return after high dose chemotherapy by hitchhiking back into the body with the stem cells (Stewart, 1996). Therefore, new methods of removing cancer cells from bone marrow or blood stem cells are urgently needed. Phototherapy (chapter 19) has been successful in killing some cancer cells in bone marrow samples (Gulati, 1994). Monoclonal antibodies (chapter 19) have also been used. Gene therapy is another possible approach. Some researchers think that treating the stem cells with the *p53* gene might kill contaminating cancer cells (Davis, 1996). *P53* can trigger apoptosis in cancer cells with DNA damage, but should not damage normal stem cells. Another possibility would be to insert the *bcl-xs* gene, another apoptosis trigger; normal bone marrow stem cells happen to be resistant to *bcl-xs* (Clarke, 1995).

Predicting the responders

It would be tremendously helpful to patients if physicians could predict who would be most likely to benefit from the high dose chemotherapy. Some patients might be spared the rigors of this treatment, if their cancer was likely to return almost as soon as with conventional treatment. On the other hand, undecided patients might be more willing to try high dose chemotherapy if they had a good chance of being cured.

Recent studies have begun to offer some clues as to who might be expected to respond well to high dose chemotherapy. Women whose cancers developed slowly and which responded, at first, to conventional treatments, seem to have the best chance of a cure. This seems to be true for both breast cancer (Vaughan, 1997; Stewart; 1996) and ovarian cancer (Stewart, 1996). In one study, researchers estimated that one fourth to one half of breast cancer patients who were in complete remission before high dose treatment, were still in remission two years after high dose therapy (Vaughan, 1997). Another source of information is the Autologous Blood and Bone Marrow Transplant Registry. They estimate that 20% of breast cancer patients who were in complete remission before high dose therapy were still alive 4 years or more after treatment without progression of the disease; 30% were still alive either with or without signs of cancer (Vaughan, 1997). Patients under 45 years old and those with estrogen receptors on their tumors also seemed to have better responses (Vaughan, 1997). Unfortunately, patients with partial remissions after conventional treatment, or unresponsive cancers, had equally poor outcomes from high dose chemotherapy (Vaughan, 1997).

There is, however, much to be done, before high dose chemotherapy with stem cell support can become a standard treatment for cancer. New ways of predicting which patients will respond are needed. Better removal of cancer cells from the stem cells is critical. The combination of high dose chemotherapy with other treatment types also seems promising. In one study, adding a cytokine called interferon gamma after treatment seemed to improve survival, perhaps helping to kill the remaining cancer cells (Stewart, 1996). In this study, 41% of patients with metastatic breast cancer treated with this combination survived at least 4 and a half years without progression of their disease, and 53% survived overall. For many patients, those might be odds worth risking.

Chapter 14

Manipulating growth factors

One benefit of basic cancer research has been a better understanding of what makes a cancer cell grow. Several of the genes we once knew only as mysterious "oncogenes" have been identified as genes for growth factors, or for their receptors (Zalutsky, 1997). Armed with this new knowledge, researchers now hope to stop those growth factor receptors from stimulating cancer cells to grow.

Growth factors are chemical messengers, sent from one cell to another, which tell the recipient to divide and make more cells. Potential recipients of the message have growth factor receptors. The growth factors attach to these receptors. Each growth factor has its own receptor (or shares a receptor with a limited number of other growth factors). For example, the fibroblast growth factor (FGF) attaches only to the FGF receptor; it cannot attach to the epidermal growth factor receptor or any other growth factor receptor. When the growth factor docks with its receptor, the receptor sends a message to the nucleus of the cell, using a series of molecules as messengers, and turns on genes for cell growth. Not all cells have receptors for all growth factors; if a growth factor is in their environment for which they have no receptor, they are simply oblivious to the message.

Many cancer cells have become greedy for growth factors. In fact, many of them have found ways to get more growth stimulation than they are entitled to. Researchers are, however, finding ways to deprive tumors of these extra growth factors, in an effort to slow tumor growth.

Inhibiting growth factor production

Some tumors produce large amounts of growth factors (Figure 14.1), which stimulate their cells and limit their need for growth factors from the rest of the body (Zumkeller, 1995). One way to suppress these growth factors is to inject extra growth factor receptors into the body (Zumkeller, 1995). These extra receptors act as decoys and can prevent the growth factors from attaching to the real receptors on cancer cells. Drugs such as suramin, which inhibits the production of several different growth factors, are also being tested (Elmajian, 1997; Zumkeller, 1995). For example, suramin is being tried for some cases of prostate cancer which do not respond to conventional treatment. (Elmajian, 1995)

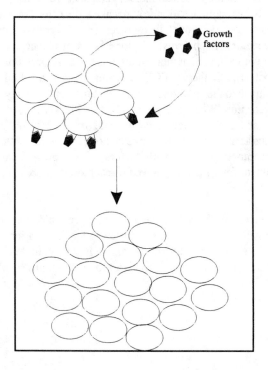

Figure 14.1 Some cancers make growth factors which stimulate their own cells to grow.

Inhibiting growth factor receptors

Cancer cells often have too many growth factor receptors, as well. Sometimes, these receptors are normal, but the increased numbers make the cancer cell oversensitive to growth factors in its environment. At other times, cancer cells make abnormal growth factor receptors which are constantly active, even when they are not attached to a growth factor (Figure 14.2). Excessive numbers of growth factor receptors on a cell, or mutated receptors, can contribute to cancers by sending constant signals to the cell to divide (Barinaga, 1997b). Important growth factor receptors in cancer treatment include the epidermal growth factor (EGF) receptor, a probable growth factor receptor known as HER-2/neu, and several other receptors.

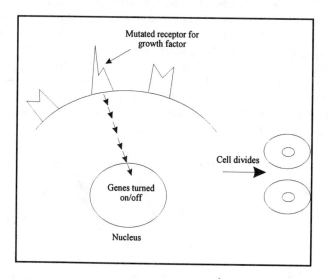

Figure 14.2. Mutated receptors can send growth signals even when no growth factor is attached.

Inhibiting the EGF and PDGF receptors

Epidermal growth factor (EGF) normally stimulates many different types of cells to grow. The EGF receptor is hyperactive in many cancers, including breast cancers, bladder cancers, and a type of brain tumor known as a glioblastoma (Zalutsky, 1997; Barinaga, 1997b). Efforts to block the EGF receptors on cancer cells and slow the growth of tumors have met with some success. One technique is to make an antibody which will stick to the growth factor receptor and block the spot where the growth factor usually docks (Figure 14.3). Any growth factor which then tries to attach to this receptor will find it already occupied. Antibodies to the EGF receptor have been able to inhibit the growth of breast cancer cells and other transplanted tumors in animals (Baselga, 1994; Dean, 1994). Antibodies to the EGF receptor have recently been tested in phase I (safety) trials in human cancer patients and appeared to be safe (Baselga, 1994). One fear with antibodies to normal proteins, such as the EGF receptor, is that they might also attach to normal cells carrying the protein, and harm them. In human safety trials, however, antibodies seemed to attach mainly to tumor cells. Recently, researchers have discovered a mutated EGF receptor which seems to be found only on tumor cells; it may be useful for aiming antibodies even more specifically to cancer cells (Zalutsky, 1997).

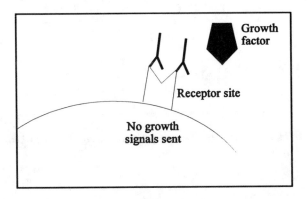

Figure 14.3. Antibodies can block growth factors from attaching to their receptor.

Antibodies have some drawbacks. They are expensive because they must be made in animals and purified, and they must be injected into the blood (Barinaga, 1997b). They are also ineffective against mutated growth factor receptors, which send growth signals without attaching to a growth factor. Investigators are, therefore, trying to find other ways to inhibit growth factor receptors inside the cells (Barinaga, 1997b). One way to do this is to manipulate some of the signals sent inside cells by growth factor receptors. For example, researchers at Sugen company (Redwood City, California) have produced a drug called Su-101, which prevents signaling from the receptor for platelet derived growth factor (PDGF). Su-101 has passed safety tests in 150 patients and has been promising against brain cancers known as a glioblastomas, whose growth is dependent on PDGF (Barinaga, 1997b). Large scale trials of Su-101 have been proposed.

Suppressing the HER-2/neu receptor

An oncogene known as *HER-2*, *neu*, or *erbB-2*, produces another growth factor receptor which may be important in cancer treatment. (This receptor is called p185HER-2, but we will just refer to it as the *HER-2* receptor, to keep from getting lost in the terminology.) Researchers are not yet certain which growth factor(s) normally attach to the HER-2 receptor (Bender MedSystems, 1998). The leading candidate is a protein known as Neu differentiation factor (or Heregulin in humans). Normally, the *HER-2/neu* gene is more active before birth than after (Disis, 1997). In adults, a few cells still make small amounts of the *HER-2* receptor, but the gene has been turned off in most cells. It has been turned back on in some cancers.

Re-activation of the *HER-2/neu* gene in adult cells seems to cause uncontrolled cell growth and contribute to the development of cancers (Bender MedSystems, 1998; Viloria Petit, 1997). In humans, the *HER-2/neu* gene is overactive in some breast, ovarian, uterine, lung, stomach and mouth cancers (Hung, 1995; Pietras, 1994; Disis, 1997). Roughly 20-40 percent of human breast cancers and 30 percent of human ovarian cancers have too many copies of the HER-2 receptor (Disis, 1997). These cancers are the ones that usually respond more poorly to treatment. Cancers which have active *HER-2/neu* genes are more likely to metastasize in animal models of cancer (Hung, 1995).This also seems to be true for humans (although there is one exception, discussed below with HER-2 vaccines).

Researchers hope that suppressing the HER-2 receptor will decrease the aggressiveness of a cancer (Hung, 1995). Some investigators have tried to tame tumors by stopping the cell from making HER-2 receptors. If, for example, the *HER-2/neu* gene can be stopped from making its messenger RNA, then no protein can be made. Coincidentally, some viruses carry genes which do just that. A virus called adenovirus-5 has a gene (called E1A) whose product can inhibit the *HER-2/neu* gene (Hung, 1995). A protein called "large T" from another virus can do the same thing (Hung, 1995). Researchers have been able to deliver E1A or large T genes into cancer cells in mice (Hung, 1995). They found that these virus proteins suppressed the growth of the tumors, and improved the survival of the mice. Clinical trials of such gene therapy are now being started in human cancer patients (Hortobagyi, 1998). Other ways to prevent the HER-2 receptor production are also being investigated. For example, one group is trying to put antibodies inside cells, to block newly made HER-2 proteins from reaching the surface of the cell (Disis, 1997).

Other investigators are trying to turn off HER-2 receptors already on the surfaces of cells. For example, antibodies to the HER-2 receptor can block its interaction with its growth factor. These antibodies have been able to suppress the growth of some tumors in mice and some humans (Pietras, 1994; Bender MedSystems, 1998). In one early study, tumors responded in five of 44 women treated with HER-2 antibodies (Barinaga, 1997b). Researchers have actually had some pleasant surprises using HER-2 antibodies. Sometimes, these antibodies seem to work better inside the body than on cancer cells grown in the laboratory (Viloria Petit, 1997). A new study suggests one reason for this. In addition to suppressing cancer cell growth, the antibodies also seem to inhibit the formation of new blood vessels in tumors (Viloria Petit, 1997). Cancer cells send messages to blood vessels to stimulate their growth; antibodies to HER-2 seem to prevent that message from being sent.

Suppressing the HER-2 receptor can also increase the effectiveness of conventional chemotherapy drugs, when these two treatments are used together (Pietras, 1994). This combination may be particularly useful against cancers that have become resistant to drugs. For example, antibodies to HER-2 can make drug-resistant cancer cells more sensitive to Cisplatin in the laboratory (Pietras, 1994). They also seem to increase the effectiveness of Cisplatin in patients. In one study, antibodies and Cisplatin helped some women whose breast cancers were no longer responsive to Cisplatin alone (Barinaga, 1997b). Tumors in nine of these 36 women responded to the treatment. Some researchers think that the HER-2 antibodies may prevent the cell from repairing DNA damage caused by the drugs (Pietras, 1994). Other researchers have suggested that the antibodies increase p53 protein in cells and make cells more likely to commit suicide (apoptosis) in response to DNA damage (Bacus, 1996). A new study has enrolled 650 women with breast cancer to test HER-2 antibodies alone, or antibodies in combination with Cisplatin; the results of this study are expected sometime in 1998 (Barinaga, 1997b).

HER-2/neu vaccines

Having too much HER-2 receptor on cancer cells, as we have mentioned, is usually a bad sign. There is, however, one exception to this. In some cases of early breast cancer, cells of the immune system have entered the tumor and seem to be responding to the HER-2 receptor (Disis, 1997). In these cases, the HER-2 receptor does not seem to be associated with a poor outlook for the patient. Some researchers, therefore, think that immune responses against the HER-2 receptor might be able to suppress some tumors. They hope to stimulate immune responses in other patients by giving them vaccines. Vaccines to HER-2 are currently being tested in humans with cancer (Disis, 1997). Animal studies suggest that such vaccines will be most effective in preventing regrowth of small tumors in patients put into remission with surgery, radiation or chemotherapy.

IGF-1 - a new association with cancer?

New research shows that men with high levels of a growth factor called insulin-like growth factor 1 (IGF-1) are four times as likely to develop prostate cancer than men with very low levels of IGF-1 (Barinaga, 1998b; Chan, 1998). IGF-1 stimulates prostate cells to grow (Barinaga, 1998b). Unpublished work by Michael Pollak and colleagues has shown that high levels of IGF-1 may also result in an increased risk for breast cancer (Barinago, 1998). Researchers are also looking for an association between this growth factor and colon cancer (Barinaga, 1998b). Some researchers speculate that lowering IGF-1 levels could decrease the risk of prostate or other cancers.

Chapter 15

Hormones and anti-hormones in cancer treatment

Some cancers can be killed by depriving them of hormones. Hormones are one of the two major communication systems in the human body (the other is the nerves).They are chemical messengers sent from glands to various organs: hormones may tell that organ to grow, or make sperm, or increase their intake of blood sugar, or any number of other activities. When hormones affect growth (cell division) in an organ, cancer cells from that organ may still be able to respond, at least partially, to the hormone. Preventing the hormone from reaching the cancer cells may be able to slow or even stop the growth of the tumor. In some cases, these cells remain dependent enough on hormones that they can actually be killed by hormone withdrawal.

Hormone manipulations have been particularly successful in cancers of the reproductive tract, such as prostate cancer and breast cancer. The organs where these cancers originate are controlled by sex hormones.

Hormone treatments in prostate cancer
The male sex hormones

Testosterone is the major sex hormone in men. Testosterone is converted into dihydrotestosterone in some cells; together, these two hormones are known as androgens. Androgens stimulate the development of the male reproductive organs at puberty and maintain them thereafter. They also help to stimulate the production of sperm. Testosterone production is controlled by a small hormone gland at the base of the brain called the pituitary gland (Figure 15.1). The pituitary gland is, in turn, controlled by the brain. When testosterone is needed, part of the brain called the hypothalamus makes a hormone, gonadotropin releasing hormone (GnRH). GnRH is sent to the pituitary gland, where it stimulates the release of two other hormones, called follicle stimulating hormone (FSH) and luteinizing hormone (LH). LH and FSH enter the blood, and eventually reach the testes. LH instructs cells in the testes to make and release testosterone. FSH and testosterone together stimulate the production of sperm.

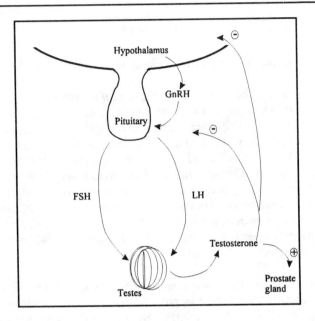

Figure 15.1. Control of testosterone production by the hypothalamus and pituitary gland.

In healthy men, testosterone production is controlled so that it neither rises too high nor falls too low. Testosterone controls the pituitary gland and brain to keep its own blood levels from becoming excessive. As the amount of testosterone in the blood increases, it suppresses the production of LH and GnRH. (Different hormones from the testes, called inhibins, turn off FSH production from the pituitary).

Inhibiting male hormones to control prostate cancer

The prostate gland is a small gland around the base of the bladder, which makes some of the fluids in semen. Prostate carcinoma is one of the most common cancers of men. It is usually a slowly growing cancer (Cerosimo, 1996) but it may spread locally to other organs, including the bladder, or eventually metastasize (Vetrovsky, 1997). Prostate cancer, like any other cancer, becomes most deadly when it metastasizes. When it is detected early, 80 percent of patients survive for at least 5 years after the diagnosis (Vetrovsky, 1997). Prostate cancers which metastasize have a much worse outlook. Ninety percent of men with metastatic prostate cancer are expected to survive for one year, but only 30 percent for three years and 10 percent for nine years (Elmajian, 1997).

If the cancer has not spread very far, surgery or radiation may be able to cure it (Vetrovsky, 1997). There are fewer options for metastatic cancers. Unfortunately, chemotherapy has not been very effective for prostate cancer (Vetrovsky, 1997; Cerosimo, 1996). Drugs which suppress the male sex hormones are, however, often very effective. Most prostate cancers will shrink at least temporarily when the androgens, testosterone and dihydrotestosterone, are suppressed (Vetrovsky, 1997). Anti-androgen treatment is often combined with surgery or radiation for localized cancers (Vetrovsky, 1997). In cases where the tumor has spread too far for surgery or radiation, or when the tumor returns after surgery, anti-androgens can be used to shrink the cancer and reduce the symptoms for a time (Vetrovsky, 1997). Unfortunately, most metastatic prostate cancers will eventually become nonresponsive to anti-androgens and begin to grow again (Elmajian, 1997). There are several different ways to suppress androgens in the body. Some of the most effective are to stop androgen production from the testes, by either surgical or medical castration.

Surgical castration

The simplest way to remove testosterone and dihydrotestosterone from the body is surgical castration, the removal of the testes (Elmajian, 1997; Vetrovsky, 1997). For some men, surgical castration has its advantages. Testosterone levels drop by more than 90 percent and most men experience relief from their symptoms almost immediately (Elmajian, 1997). It is also considerably less expensive than the alternatives (Elmajian, 1997). Not surprisingly, not all men feel comfortable with this option. There is, however, an alternative: androgen levels can be suppressed with drugs. This is known as medical castration.

Medical castration - estrogen and GnRH mimics

Medical castration is the reduction of androgen levels with drugs (Elmajian, 1997; Vetrovsky, 1997). This treatment is not permanent, and it does not involve surgical removal of the testes. One older type of medical castration is to give the man a form of estrogen, the female sex hormone (Elmajian, 1997). Estrogen, like testosterone, suppresses LH and GnRH in the pituitary and brain (Elmajian, 1997). Once LH and GnRH are turned down, they can no longer stimulate testosterone production and testosterone levels will drop. Unfortunately, some of these estrogen drugs, such as diethylstilbestrol, increase the risk of blood clots forming in the circulation, and the risk of a stroke or heart attack (Elmajian, 1997).

Newer synthetic drugs which mimic GnRH have fewer serious side effects than estrogen and are being increasingly used as medical castration. They include the drugs leuprolide (Leuprorelin) and goserelin (Zoladex) (Elmajian, 1997). At first, it might seem very odd, and counterproductive, to be using drugs which mimic GnRH. But these drugs suppress androgens by an indirect route. The GnRH mimicking drugs will cause a sudden rise in LH and testosterone; the excess testosterone then turns down the GnRH receptors in the pituitary and LH receptors in the testes (Elmajian, 1997). Essentially, the system sees an overload of testosterone, which stimulates it to make everything less sensitive to GnRH. Eventually, testosterone decreases. Unfortunately, that first surge of testosterone can make tumor metastasis grow (Elmajian, 1997). For this reason, a treatment which more directly suppresses testosterone production is given during the first part of the treatment (Elmajian, 1997).

Recently, a large study tested whether adding goserelin to radiation treatment had any advantage over radiation alone. In this study, goserelin did increase survival and reduce disease (Bolla, 1997). Seventy nine percent of patients treated with goserelin were free of disease for at least five years after treatment; only 62 percent of those treated with radiation alone had no signs of cancer at five years.

Drugs that block testosterone effects

Some new anti-androgens, such as Flutamide, bicalutamide and Nilutamide, are not designed to lower androgen levels in the blood; instead, they prevent the existing testosterone from stimulating prostate cancer cells (Elmajian, 1997). Androgens, like all hormones, must first attach to a cell's receptors before they can affect that cell. These drugs attach themselves to the receptor, instead, and prevent the androgens from reaching it. These drugs have fewer side effects than drugs which lower testosterone levels.

Unfortunately, Flutamide and its relatives cannot completely block the effects of the androgens (Elmajian, 1997). They are, therefore, rarely effective alone. They are, however, often used in combination with either surgical or medical castration. This might seem a little redundant, since testosterone levels are already being suppressed by the castration. As much as 10 percent of the androgens in the blood are, however, actually made by the adrenal glands (2 small glands above the kidneys) (Elmajian, 1997). Androgens from the adrenals are not influenced by LH or GnRH, and so they cannot be decreased by either medical or surgical castration. Flutamide and related drugs, however, can block these androgens from acting on the cancer cells. In two studies, they increased the survival of patients with metastatic prostate cancer by 7 months; however, in other experiments, they were not beneficial (Elmajian, 1997; Brogden, 1995). Other clinical trials are in progress (Elmajian, 1997).

One odd fact is that sometimes, when a patient is on Flutamide and the cancer returns, stopping the Flutamide may actually improve the symptoms (Elmajian, 1997). A possible explanation is that the androgen

receptors in the cancer cells actually mutate, so that they treat Flutamide as they would testosterone (Elmajian, 1997). Now, instead of sitting harmlessly in the cell, the Flutamide/receptor combination stimulates prostate cells, just as testosterone would have!

Finasteride lowers testosterone activity in cells

Although we usually think of testosterone when we think of male sex hormones, dihydrotestosterone is actually a stronger androgen than testosterone. In fact, enzymes convert testosterone to dihydrotestosterone in some cells (Hong, 1997). A new drug, Finasteride, stops these enzymes and prevents this conversion. In essence, it lowers the activity of the male sex hormones. Finasteride is being considered for the treatment of early prostate cancer, and for prostate cancer prevention (chapter 28).

Androgen sensitivity may be a predictor of prostate cancer

One interesting recent discovery is that different forms of the androgen receptor molecule, which turns on genes in the prostate gland in response to testosterone and other male sex hormones, may influence a man's likelihood of getting prostate cancer (Anon, 1996). The gene for this receptor molecule contains a base sequence CAG, repeated several times. In different men, the number of repeats may vary from 11 to 33. With fewer repeats, a stronger signal is transmitted to the genes - and a stronger signal is associated with a higher risk of prostate cancer.

Hormone treatments in breast cancer
The female hormones

The female sex hormones are estrogens and progesterone. The control of these hormones is quite similar to the control of androgens. (This is not so surprising when we realize that, during development of a baby, the reproductive organs develop from a set of organs which are identical in males and females until the seventh week.) The hypothalamus also makes GnRH in women and sends it to the pituitary, where it stimulates the release of FSH and LH. LH and FSH stimulate the development of eggs and the production of estrogens and progesterone from the ovaries. There are several natural estrogens in the body, including estradiol, estrone, and estriol. The estrogens stimulate the female reproductive organs, including the breasts, to grow at puberty.

The control of estrogen and progesterone levels is similar to (but a little more complex than) the control of androgens in men. Estrogen turns off LH and GnRH secretion, except just before the release of an egg from the ovary (when it actually stimulates a burst of LH production). In general, a moderate and steady level of circulating estrogen inhibits LH production.

One difference between men and women is that, in women, the ovaries eventually stop making estrogen and progesterone. (In men, testosterone production does not stop.) This event, called menopause, can affect some of the hormone treatments used for breast cancer.

Inhibiting estrogens in breast cancers

Normal cells from the breast have receptors for estrogen. Some breast cancer cells have also kept their estrogen receptors. Treatments which block estrogen are effective in roughly 30 percent of women with breast cancer (Hortobagyi, 1995). Early in the disease, hormonal treatments can help to cure the cancer; in advanced disease, they are used to prolong survival or reduce the symptoms (Vogel, 1996). The most common hormone treatments for breast cancer are anti-estrogens. Anti-estrogens are only effective in cancers which have retained their estrogen receptors. The most commonly used anti-estrogenic drug is Tamoxifen.

Tamoxifen

In breast cancer cells, estrogen attaches to a receptor inside the cell; the estrogen/receptor complex is then transported to the nucleus and turns on genes for cell growth. Tamoxifen attaches to the estrogen receptor and blocks it from interacting with estrogen (Kennemans, 1996). The Tamoxifen/receptor complex has different effects in different cells (Figure 15.2). In breast cells, it seems to be inactive; it simply prevents estrogen from stimulating the cell. In the bone, cardiovascular system, liver and uterus, however, Tamoxifen acts just like estrogen (Kennemans, 1996). In the bone, this is beneficial: both estrogen and Tamoxifen help to maintain strong bones. In the cardiovascular system, like estrogen, Tamoxifen can protect against heart disease. In the uterus, however, it can promote the growth of cells and seems to increase the risk of uterine cancer. The risk of uterine cancers increased two to six-fold during long-term Tamoxifen use, in some studies (Kennemans, 1996; Wilking, 1997; Marshall, 1998). In one study, researchers may have also seen an increase in colon and stomach cancers (Kennemans, 1996). In animal experiments, Tamoxifen also increased liver cancer (liver cells have estrogen receptors), but it does not appear to have this effect in humans (Kennemans, 1996; Wilking, 1997).

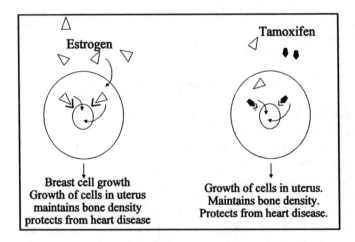

Figure 15.2. Comparison of estrogen and Tamoxifen.

More than half of advanced breast cancers which have estrogen receptors respond to Tamoxifen (Wilking, 1997). Tamoxifen has been estimated to decrease the death rate from breast cancer by 25% (Kennemans, 1996). In fact, there is some question whether giving chemotherapy drugs with Tamoxifen to maintain a remission actually has any advantage over simply giving Tamoxifen alone (Vogel, 1996). It even has some benefit in metastatic breast cancers, where a chance of a cure is often very poor.

In one clinical trial, 14% (of 156) patients with metastatic breast cancer had complete remissions with Tamoxifen; tumors shrunk partially in another 6% (Kuss, 1997).

One complicating factor with Tamoxifen therapy is that it can have different effects in women before and after menopause. Tamoxifen decreases estrogen in post-menopausal women, but is actually capable of increasing estrogen levels in premenopausal women (Kennemans, 1996). Therefore, doctors may suggest alternative treatments, such as removal of the ovaries, in younger breast cancer patients(Vogel, 1996). Experiments are being conducted to compare Tamoxifen (combined with other hormonal treatments) to removal of the ovaries in pre-menopausal women (Vogel, 1996). Tamoxifen has also been recently tested as a cancer preventative (chapter 28).

Newer anti-estrogens

Because Tamoxifen may increase cancers of the uterus, and possibly other cancers, newer anti-estrogens are being developed and tested. Raloxifene, for example, is similar to Tamoxifen, but it does not seem to promote cancers of the uterus (Pennisi, 1996a; Hong, 1997). Like Tamoxifen, Raloxifene acts like estrogen in the bones, which would help to preserve bone density (Pennisi, 1996a; Hong, 1997). Raloxifene is already in use as a drug in humans; it is used to prevent osteoporosis in women. It may be effective in breast cancer treatment, but it has not yet been thoroughly evaluated (Hong, 1997). Other drugs which have no estrogen effects in the uterus have also been developed and are been tested in preclinical and clinical trials (Kennemans, 1996). One drug, called LY353381, has been shown to prevent breast cancer in animals and appears to be more potent than Raloxifene (Hong, 1997).

Aromatase inhibitors

A second way to inhibit estrogens is to block their production. Blocking enzymes called aromatases can decrease the amount of estrogens in the body (Brodie, 1994). Aromatase inhibitors, such as ARIMIDEX, vorazole, and letrozole, are being tested as estrogen inhibitors in breast cancer patients (Brodie, 1994; Plourde, 1995). In human phase I (safety) studies, they could decrease estrogen to undetectable levels in breast cancer patients (Plourde, 1995). Seventeen of the patients from this study have been using aromatase inhibitors for more than 20 months, with no serious side effects. There have been some promising clinical responses in these patients, and phase II studies are underway. In another study, an aromatase inhibitor was given to 240 breast cancer patients who had relapsed after taking Tamoxifen (Brodie, 1994). In 26 percent of these patients, their cancers regressed to some extent and, in another 25 percent, the cancer stopped growing and did not progress for a time. In one clinical trial, patients who had never taken Tamoxifen had similar responses to Tamoxifen or aromatase inhibitors (Brodie, 1994). In these patients, 33 percent of the cancers regressed with aromatase inhibitors and 37 percent with Tamoxifen treatment.

Estrogen to make breast cancer cells sensitive to drugs

One unusual, but seemingly risky, idea has been to use estrogen to stimulate breast cancer cells into growth, to enhance killing by drugs which can only kill actively dividing cells. In a small pilot study, 3 human breast cancers in mice were first treated with estrogen to stimulate growth, then with mitomycin C to kill the actively dividing cells (Oka, 1996). This treatment resulted in increased effectiveness of the mitomycin C. While intriguing, this idea remains to be further tested for safety!

Chapter 16

Vitamins in cancer treatment

For years, researchers have known that a diet high in certain fruits and vegetables can reduce the risk of some cancers (Sankaranaryanan, 1996; Gaziano, 1996).Yet attempts to tease out the exact ingredients in these foods has been difficult; the factor, or combination of factors, seems to be rather elusive. Many researchers think that the important cancer-fighting agents may be vitamins, particularly the antioxidant vitamins (which prevent cell damage by mopping up free radicals). In chapter 28, we will discuss a number of studies designed to prevent cancer with vitamins. In some cases, however, vitamins may also be useful for cancer treatment.

Vitamin A, beta-carotene, and the retinoids

Vitamin A (retinol) and related chemicals called carotenoids and retinoids may turn out to be some of the more effective vitamins for cancer treatment and prevention. Vitamin A is found in fish oils, liver, egg yolks, butter and cream (Berkow, 1992). It can be quite toxic when too much of it is eaten: among other problems, it can cause severe headaches, vomiting weakness, skin problems and birth defects (Berkow, 1992). Vitamin A can also, however, be made in the human body from beta carotene and other carotenoids, which are found in yellow and leafy green vegetables (Berkow, 1992). Carotenoids don't seem to cause obvious problems when eaten in excess, except sometimes to give a deep yellow tinge to the skin (Berkow, 1992). In the body, vitamin A is converted into several chemicals called retinoids.

The retinoids seem to be important during development in the embryo (Cornic, 1994). They also stimulate some cells in adults to differentiate (Cornic, 1994; Sankaranaryanan, 1996). Differentiation (Figure 16.1) is the process where a cell turns into a normal mature cell of its type; in a sense, differentiation is when a cell "grows up." When new cells are made, they have few special skills; in fact, they look rather primitive and nondescript. During differentiation, these new cells change their appearance, develop new functions, and eventually, turn into mature cells.

Muscle cells, for example, develop the ability to contract. The more differentiated a cell is, the less likely it is to undergo cell division. By stimulating differentiation, therefore, retinoids can suppress cell division.

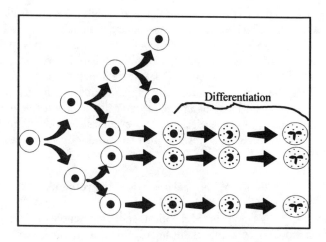

Figure 16.1. Most of the cells produced by a normal dividing cell eventually differentiate. A few remain undifferentiated and can continue to make new cells.

The retinoids seem to be some of the more promising drugs in vitamin therapy of cancer (Cornic, 1994). In particular, retinoids have found a valuable niche for the treatment of a type of leukemia called acute promyelocytic leukemia. Acute promyelocytic leukemia is a cancer of the bone marrow cells which produce granulocytes (a type of white blood cell). Retinoic acid, a retinoid, can force these leukemia cells to differentiate into normal mature-looking granulocytes (Cornic, 1994). In the process, these granulocytes, like normal granulocytes, lose their ability to divide. In fact, a normal granulocyte has a very short lifespan, measured in days; therefore, retinoic acid essentially stimulates these cancer cells to die. In clinical trials, 80 percent of patients with acute promyelocytic leukemia who took retinoic acid had complete remission of their cancer (Cornic, 1994).

Retinoid treatment may be so successful in this cancer because the cells often have a mutation in a retinoic acid receptor. In many of these patients, one chromosome has broken and has been attached to another chromosome at a specific location (Cornic, 1994). This process creates a mutant gene which contains a gene for a retinoic acid receptor joined to another gene called *PML* (Cornic, 1994). The protein made from this mutant gene seems to end up in a different place in the nucleus than the normal protein; somehow, this change in location then blocks cell differentiation (Lavau, 1994). Some researchers speculate that, when the mutant protein is located in the wrong parts of the nucleus, critical molecules in differentiation follow it and don't do their job properly (Lavau, 1994). Retinoic acid somehow seems to force this wandering protein back into its proper location (Lavau, 1994).

Unfortunately, retinoids have not been as successful against most advanced cancers (Sankaranaryanan, 1996).They have not been able to decrease the death rate from cancers of the stomach and esophagus (Sankaranaryanan, 1996). They have also been ineffective in treating skin cancers which return after the initial treatment (Sankaranaryanan, 1996). And, although retinoic acid could cause changes in the appearance of melanoma cells in the laboratory, neither it nor another retinoid could slow the growth of the cells (Prasad, 1994). Retinoids are, however, still being tested in other types of cancer. For example, retinoids, or drugs which increase the levels of retinoids in the body, are being considered as treatments for prostate cancer and are in clinical trials (Elmajian, 1997). They also seem to be promising in cancer prevention (chapter 28).

Vitamins C and E and the carotenoids

There seems to be little evidence that vitamin C is a good treatment for existing cancers, although it is being investigated as a cancer preventative (chapter 28). For example, an analysis of existing experiments by the National Cancer Institute concluded that vitamin C does not seem to be effective in the treatment of established cancers (National Cancer Institute, 1997b). In some animal models of cancer, vitamin C did seem to increase the activity of other drugs against cancer or protected animals against the side effects of those drugs. In other animal studies, however, there seemed to be no benefit. In studies of advanced cancers in humans, vitamin C did not seem to be beneficial.

A few recent studies suggest that vitamin E compounds may be able to suppress or kill cancer cells grown in the laboratory (Turley, 1997; Yu, 1997). In general, vitamin E seems to have been investigated more as a cancer preventative (chapter 28) than as a cancer treatment. There is, however, an intriguing study on the effects of a mixture of natural compounds and vitamin E for the treatment of skin cancers. This recent study investigated the effects of a compound known as Roidex, a blend of squalene (a chemical related to cholesterol), vitamin E and aloe vera, in skin tumors in mice (Desai, 1996). Without Roidex, 3 percent of the tumors spontaneously regressed (1 of 29 mice had a spontaneous regression). In the mice treated with Roidex, however, a third of the mice (13 of 39) had regression of their tumors. Roidex also slightly decreased the development of new skin tumors: tumors developed in 33 percent of the mice not treated with Roidex, and 27 percent of the mice treated with Roidex. Researchers do not yet know what chemical in this mixture was responsible for the cancer regressions.

Chapter 17

Stopping cancer cells from spreading -
prevention of metastasis

One fact becomes very obvious if you browse the literature on cancer: localized cancers can be scary but are often quite treatable, but metastatic cancers or cancers which rapidly invade surrounding tissues are deadly. For example the American Cancer Society (1998) estimates the 5 year survival rate for patients with localized breast cancer at 97 percent, for breast cancer with regional spread at 76 percent, and for breast cancer with distant metastasis at 21 percent Some new cancer drugs are being developed specifically to prevent metastasis.

How cancer cells metastasize

Cancer cell metastasis begins when a cell or small group of cells acquires the ability to move. Ordinarily, only a few normal cells (such as the cells of the immune system) regularly travel around the body. Most cells lose their mobility after they move to their final positions in the body before birth. They become tightly attached to their neighbors and to their surroundings, and stop making the proteins necessary for movement. Cancer cells, however, are not so sedentary. Many of them develop characteristics which give them the ability to move. They stick less tightly to neighboring cells than normal (Dickson, 1996). The stickiness of other molecules, which help the cancer cell crawl along surfaces, may increase (Dickson, 1996). A cancer cell can also become capable of dissolving obstacles in its path (Dickson, 1996). Finally, with all of these abilities, a cancer cell can crawl away from the tumor, dissolving the barriers before it. At this stage, a tumor is considered to be "locally invasive"; the tumor is spreading and infiltrating normal surrounding tissues.

Some invading cancer cells reach and enter blood vessels or lymphatic vessels; these cells can metastasize to distant parts of the body. Cells which enter lymphatic vessels are swept to nearby lymph nodes in the lymph fluid. Lymph nodes are usually the first place surgeons look to find metastatic cells. Cancer cells also leave the tumor in blood vessels.

Researchers think that the new blood vessels inside tumors are very important to cancer metastasis. In particular, the strange and leaky blood vessels inside tumors may make it particularly easy for tumor cells to invade the blood (Hall, 1995; Dickson, 1996). Cancer cells can also move from lymphatic vessels to blood vessels (Figure 17.1), or blood vessels to lymph nodes (Cheville, 1983).. Once it is inside a blood vessel, a cancer cell is swept along until it lodges somewhere. Often, it is trapped in a small blood vessel feeding an organ. Most metastatic cells do not survive, but those which do can grow and generate a new tumor (Cheville, 1983). Organs which often contain metastasis include the lungs, liver, bone, lymph nodes, kidney and brain (Cheville, 1983).

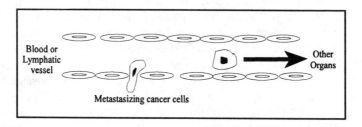

Figure 17.1. Metastasizing cancer cells squeeze through the walls of a blood or lymphatic vessel and are carried in the fluid to other organs.

Preventing metastasis

The complexity of the metastatic process means that there may be many ways to prevent metastasis and local invasion. Increasing the stickiness of the cells might help to glue them into place. Preventing their ability to dissolve barriers might put roadblocks into their path. Preventing the formation of new blood vessels inside the tumor (chapter 18) would reduce their chances of finding a blood vessel that they could get into. Other drugs might decrease their ability to survive in the blood and divide at new sites. Metastasis suppression is still in its infancy, but, slowly, scientists are discovering some of the genes and proteins involved in invasion. There is, however, much to be done yet, and we will find only a few answers and hints, and a few new drugs.

Sticky proteins and cancer cells

Researchers are slowly learning about the genes that make cells stick to each other and to their environment. At the moment, their findings are mainly used to predict which cancers will be more invasive or likely to metastasize. At some point in the future, however, new treatments could also come from this research.

As cells turn into cancer cells, they stick less tightly to other cells (Dickson, 1996). Some proteins which glue cells together seem to be lost from invasive cancers. Two examples are the cadherins and the product of a gene called *nm23*. Cadherin molecules attach cells to each other, suppress their movement, and promote their differentiation (Dickson, 1996). One of the cadherins, E cadherin, is lost from some breast cancer cells (Dickson, 1996). Cells which have lost E cadherin move more actively and are more invasive than cells which have normal amounts of E cadherin (Dickson, 1996). The product of *nm23* may also be involved in adhesion between cells (Parhar, 1995). Researchers know very little about *nm23*, except that it seems to be able to suppress metastasis and decreases as cells become more invasive (Dickson, 1996; Parhar, 1995). For example, putting the *nm23* gene back into cancer cells seems to suppress their ability to invade and to metastasize. Mice injected with *nm23*-modified tumor cells live longer than mice injected with unmodified cells (Parhar, 1995).

Other types of sticky proteins seem to increase in invasive cancers. Some of them probably help cancer cells adhere more tightly to components of their environment. Cancer cells can't "swim" through a fluid; they must migrate laboriously, essentially crawling along a surface. They pull themselves along by attaching and detaching their outer membranes. A cancer cell, therefore, may need increased amounts of proteins which help it to stick to certain surfaces. For example, the BEHAB protein, found in very invasive brain cancers called gliomas, seems to be involved in attaching cancer cells to a substance called hyaluronan (Barinaga, 1997c). BEHAB is found in invasive gliomas, but not in non-invasive gliomas. Breast and colon cancers may produce more of a protein which attaches to a different molecule, laminin, as they become more aggressive (Dickson, 1996).

A protein that helps cancer cells squeeze through tight spaces?

One newly discovered protein, found in some brain cancers, may help invasion in a different way. This protein makes a channel, or hole in the cell's outer membrane, which lets certain atoms (chloride ion and others) pass through (Barinaga, 1997c). The percentage of cells which have the channel increases as the cancer becomes more invasive. No one really knows the function of this channel protein yet; however, some researchers speculate that it might help the cell lose fluid so it can squeeze through tight spaces during movement. Researchers hope eventually to use this channel to treat cancers. For example, the channels might be targeted with chemicals which carry radioactive molecules to the cancers (Barinaga, 1997c).

Putting up barriers to movement

One of the most successful ways to block metastasis is to physically trap cancer cells at their origins. Fortunately for this approach, the body is a rather cluttered place. A network of tangled fibers and proteins, called the extracellular matrix, fills the spaces between organized groups of cells. To move around in this tangled web, a cell must make enzymes to clear a space in front of it as it migrates. Drugs to inhibit these enzymes are some of the most studied metastasis inhibitors (Dickson, 1996).

One of the most important proteins in the extracellular matrix is collagen. Collagen forms tough little interconnecting threads that give tissues their strength - but that can also block cell movement. Many cancer cells need enzymes to break down collagen, before they can move (Dickson, 1996). These enzymes, called matrix metalloproteinases (or collagenases), can be blocked by drugs. One new drug known as Batimastat (BB-94) inhibits a variety of metalloproteinases. (Dickson, 1996). It has been promising in mice and is being tested in humans. In one study, mice with human breast cancers were given Batimastat after surgical removal of their main tumor (Sledge, 1995). The mice treated with Batimastat had fewer metastasis and less regrowth of the original tumor than mice not given the drug. Batimastat has also been successful in mice with ovarian cancers (Dickson, 1996)

Phase I (safety) trials with Batimastat in humans are underway in the United States and Europe (Dickson, 1996). So far, some patients seem to have responded to the drug, and researchers have not seen major side effects. A new drug known as Bryostatin-1 also inhibits metalloproteinase production and cell invasiveness (Dickson, 1996). Bryostatin-1 has been able to prevent metastasis in mice with melanomas and other tumors. Phase I trials with Bryostatin 1 have been done in Europe and the drug appears to be relatively safe (Dickson, 1996).

Another enzyme, urokinase, may also be important in breaking down barriers to migration. Very invasive brain tumors, for example, have increased amounts of urokinase or related enzymes (Go, 1997). Cisplatin, one of the drugs often used to treat these tumors, may be effective partly because it inhibits urokinase and prevents the spread of the cells (Go, 1997). New ways to prevent urokinase activity or production are being investigated. For example, anti-urokinase peptides, small pieces of proteins which block urokinase, suppress metastasis (Dickson, 1996). The retinoids (chapter 16) may also be able to turn off urokinase production (Dickson, 1996).

Becoming far travelers: moving from local invasion to metastasis

Researchers do not yet know how cancer cells switch from being locally invasive to becoming metastatic (Dickson, 1996). Although the trigger for this event is likely to be in the genes, no specific gene has been identified yet. The HER2/neu receptor (chapter 14) seems to be at least indirectly involved in metastasis (Dickson, 1996). Growth factors which promote motility, such as "autocrine motility factor/AMF" and other growth factors may also be involved (Dickson, 1996).

Preventing establishment of metastatic cells

Drugs are also being developed to prevent the survival and growth of metastatic cells which have already left the main tumor and entered the blood. One way to stop these cells may be to prevent them from sticking to each other in the bloodstream. Researchers have discovered that clumps of cancer cells seem to survive and grow better than single cells (Cheville, 1993; Dickson, 1996). This may be because a single cell is less likely to be trapped in a small blood vessel somewhere, and given the opportunity to migrate into the tissue. Some researchers, therefore, are trying to force metastatic cells to travel as single cells, in the hope that these cells will die in the bloodstream.

Some cancer cells in the blood may use blood clotting proteins to stick to each other (Dickson, 1996). During blood clotting, cell fragments called platelets begin a process that ends in the formation of a sticky, tangled lattice of proteins. Ordinarily, this sticky web traps blood cells and stops bleeding. Cancer cells, however, may also use some of those sticky proteins to form clumps. Some cancer drugs may, therefore, be able to prevent metastasis by decreasing blood clotting. Cicaprost, for example, is a drug which blocks metastasis of some tumors in mice, possibly by preventing platelet activity (Dickson, 1996). Disintegrins are proteins from snake venom which can prevent cells from interacting with each other and with the extracellular matrix (Dickson, 1996). Contortrostatin is a disintegrin which stops platelets from sticking to each other. It can prevent metastasis in experimental models, probably by preventing cancer cells from sticking to each other.

There is yet one more way to stop or slow metastasis. In the next chapter, we will see how stopping blood vessel growth kills some cancer cells. Keep in mind that it can also slow metastasis by giving invasive cancer cells fewer chances to enter a blood vessel.

Chapter 18

Cutting off the supply lines - attacking normal cells to destroy the tumor

When cancer strikes, there is a natural tendency to focus on the abnormal cells themselves, and concentrate all of our scientific resources on directly destroying them. But perhaps it would be wise to remember that cancers interact with the normal cells surrounding them. Cancer cells stimulate the growth of blood vessels into the tumor and change the architecture of the normal cells and fibers surrounding the tumor. Some cancer researchers speculate that these normal tissues may be easier to attack than the cancer cells themselves, since they do not mutate and cannot as easily resist treatments designed to kill them. In a way, it's like weakening an army by cutting off its supply lines. Most of this work has been done with the blood vessels that feed tumors.

Blood vessels and tumor death

All cells need certain substances such as oxygen and nutrients to survive and grow. They also must get rid of waste products, such as carbon dioxide, to prevent being poisoned by them. Cancer cells may be very different than normal cells in many ways, but they have not lost these basic requirements for life. If they receive no food or no oxygen, or if they cannot get rid of their wastes, they die.

The movement of oxygen, nutrients, and waste products is limited by distance. Organisms which are only a few cells thick don't need blood vessels: all of the necessary substances can easily reach each cell from the outside world. But once an animal starts forming organs and tissues, it needs a way to transport the necessary substances to within a short distance of the cells. Blood in blood vessels serves that purpose. It is a lifeline to all of the cells in the body. Cut off the blood supply to any group of cells, and they will die.

A tumor is no different. When it first forms, the few cancer cells don't need a blood supply; they can get along fine with nutrients from the blood vessels already in the area. But as the tumor grows, and the mass of cells thickens, so its need for new blood vessels increases. The cells in the center of the tumor would die without a blood supply. To prevent this, the tumor cells make chemicals which signal to the body that new blood vessels are needed in the area; in response, the cells of nearby blood vessels begin to divide and grow into the developing cancer. As the cancer grows, the blood vessels grow with it. The development of these new blood vessels is called angiogenesis. Researchers have shown that, at least for some cancers, the greater the number of blood vessels in a tumor, the worse the outlook is for the patient (Craft, 1994).

Although the idea that cancers need blood vessels seems obvious today, at one time it was a radical notion. It can be traced back to the 1970's and Judah Folkman of Harvard Medical Center (Barinaga, 1997a). Folkman suggested that, if new blood vessels inside a tumor could be prevented from forming, then the cancer could no longer grow. Folkman's persistence has paid off. A whole host of new angiogeneses inhibiting drugs are in development and some of them show remarkable promise.

What makes blood vessels grow (or stop growing)

To understand the new angiogenesis inhibitors, we must first understand the signals that make blood vessels grow or stop growing. New blood vessel development, like the growth of other cells in the body, is stimulated by growth factors. For blood vessels, there seem to be many growth factors: vascular endothelial growth factor (VEGF), platelet derived endothelial cell growth factor (PDGF), basic fibroblast growth factor (FGF), transforming growth factor beta 1 (TGFβ 1) and several others (Bikfalvi, 1995; Jendraschak, 1996; Harris, 1996; Dickson, 1996). These growth factors are made either by the cancer cells themselves, or by other cells which have been stimulated by the cancer cells. The growth factors attach to receptors on the cells of blood vessels, called endothelial cells. This interaction stimulates the endothelial cells to divide. They also begin to migrate into the tumor, using enzymes to dissolve away barriers in their path (Jendraschak, 1996). Eventually, they form a network of complete new blood vessels inside the tumor. The body also has ways to stop angiogenesis. If growth factors are removed, the endothelial cells will stop dividing and forming new blood vessels. Growth inhibitory molecules may also be able to override the effects of the growth factors (Barinaga, 1997a; Jendraschak, 1996). Researchers are, therefore, looking at two obvious ways to stop angiogenesis in tumors: neutralize the growth factors, or add a growth inhibitor. An alternative may be to stop blood vessel growth by preventing the endothelial cells from moving into the tumor.

Neutralizing growth factors and other growth stimulants

Theoretically, there are several ways to successfully neutralize the growth factors for endothelial cells. Drugs might act on the cells that produce growth factors and prevent their manufacture or release. A drug could also clamp itself onto existing growth factors and physically prevent them from attaching to their receptor. Finally, a drug could attach to the receptors, and block the growth factors from getting near them. Some of these drugs are very close to becoming an option for cancer patients.

The easiest drugs to make are those which physically block the growth factors from interacting with their receptors. Several companies are, in fact, developing such drugs to stop the growth factors VEGF and basic FGF (Barinaga, 1997a). Essentially, these drugs are antibodies or other molecules which grab hold of either VEGF, basic FGF or their receptors and prevent them from stimulating the endothelial cells. Some of these drugs have been able to slow or stop cancer growth in mice, and may soon enter clinical trials (Barinaga, 1997a). In some cases, however, they may have better effects when they are injected directly into tumors than into the blood (Coppola, 1997). This may, at least for now, limit their use to tumors which are large enough to detect and accessible enough to stick a needle into.

Blocking the manufacture of growth factors does not seem to be quite as easy as preventing them from interacting with their targets. For example, the drug suramin can suppress growth factor production, but is quite toxic. A group of newer, less toxic, drugs related to suramin is being readied for clinical trials and may be more promising (Harris, 1996).

Natural blood vessel growth inhibitors

There are also several growth inhibitors, found naturally in the body, which can suppress blood vessel growth and have potential for cancer treatment. The angiopectins, for example, are naturally occurring molecules which suppress endothelial cell growth (Barinaga, 1997a). There is also a remarkable new group of angiogenesis inhibitors which are actually made by the tumor cells themselves. Physicians and cancer researchers have known for years that, when the main tumor is removed, the metastasis from that tumor will sometimes suddenly start to grow (Barinaga, 1997a). It is as if the presence of the main tumor were somehow repressing the metastasis. In the 1980's, researchers discovered that some cancer cells make angiogenesis inhibitors which suppress blood vessel growth in metastasis (Barinaga, 1997a). One puzzle is, of course, why these inhibitors only suppress blood vessels in distant metastasis, and not the main tumor itself. One idea is that, near the main tumor, there are so many growth factors that the inhibitors are overwhelmed, and blood vessels grow; farther away, however, there are fewer growth factors and the inhibitors keep vessels from growing (Barinaga, 1997a).

Researchers are naturally excited about the potential for these natural inhibitors in cancer treatment. One of these angiogenesis inhibitors, Thrombospondin, can make endothelial cells stop responding to all of the growth stimulators that have been tried so far (Barinaga, 1997a). Thrombospondin has been able to stop melanomas from metastasizing to the lungs of mice. It can also decrease the ability of breast cancer cells to stimulate blood vessel growth. Angiostatin is another inhibitor which is able to shrink tumors in mice remarkably, from 400 mg to microscopic size (Barinaga, 1997a). A third inhibitor, Endostatin, can also shrink a variety of tumors in mice ; tumors reduced by Endostatin remain small as long as the mouse receives the drug (Barinaga, 1997a). Remarkably, no resistance to Endostatin has ever seemed to develop in mice. When the mice were taken off the drug, the tumor returned; when they were again given Endostatin, the tumors regressed again. Clinical trials of Thrombospondin, Endostatin, and Angiostatin are expected to be a few years away and no one is sure yet that they will be as effective in humans as in mice (Barinaga, 1997a). If, however, they live up to their promise, they might turn out to be marvelous new tools for cancer treatment.

Putting up barriers to movement

There is another way to keep new blood vessels from forming. This is to simply block the stimulated endothelial cells from migrating into the tumor. Like other migrating cells, endothelial cells clear a path for themselves with enzymes, and blocking those enzymes may be able to stop the cell from moving. (Barinaga, 1997a).

A host of other mysterious inhibitors, including the notorious drug Thalidomide

Finally, there is a whole collection of other angiogenesis inhibitors. In fact, we don't yet know how some of them work; we only know that they do work. Both Fumagillin, a chemical made by a fungus, and platelet factor 4, made by blood cells, inhibit angiogenesis and tumor growth in mice and are entering clinical trials (Barinaga, 1997a). The most unusual and unexpected angiogenesis inhibitor, however, is the notorious tranquilizer Thalidomide (Barinaga, 1997a). Thalidomide was taken by many women in the 1960s for morning sickness. At the time, it was thought to be safe in pregnant women. It wasn't. Thalidomide resulted in the tragic birth of babies without arms or legs before this unexpected side effect was discovered and it was withdrawn from use. Now, in a bizarre twist, Thalidomide may turn out to be a new cancer treatment. Judah Folkman and his colleagues have discovered that Thalidomide is not only a tranquilizer; it is also an angiogenesis inhibitor (Barinaga, 1997a). This finding may at least partially explain the birth defects: without blood vessels, the arms and legs could not form during a baby's development.

No one is, of course, suggesting that Thalidomide be used in pregnant women. But most cancer drugs are already so toxic that pregnancy would be a guaranteed disaster when they are given. Oddly enough, considering its history, Thalidomide might turn out to be a relatively safe angiogenesis inhibitor.

Pitfalls, problems and an interesting idea for therapy

If you think about the blood vessels in cancers and in normal organs, you may already have realized that there is one problem with angiogenesis inhibitors: they stop the growth of normal endothelial cells. Although the physical structure of blood vessels in tumors is very odd, the cells making up those blood vessels are normal cells which have migrated in from normal blood vessels. So what is to prevent angiogenesis inhibitors from destroying new blood vessels forming elsewhere in the body? The answer is that, in many or most cases, they do destroy other new blood vessels as well. Usually, however, the only areas with major amounts of new blood vessel growth are the tumor and any areas of wound healing in the body. Therefore, angiogenesis inhibitors should be relatively safe for short-term use in patients without new wounds.

One problem is, however, that angiogenesis inhibitors may turn out to be a long term drug. As the experiments with Endostatin show, tumors can return when the drug is withdrawn (Barinaga, 1997a). The reason is undoubtedly that, once the tumor has shrunk to a small enough size (less than 1 to 2 mm), the blood vessels are no longer necessary to maintain the cells (Barinaga, 1997a). A nucleus of cancer cells remains, ready to grow again, once the angiogenesis inhibitor is removed. The solution may be to combine angiogenesis inhibitors with other cancer treatments. With luck, angiogenesis inhibitors would be able to shrink the tumors, so that chemotherapy, radiation or other treatments would be able to destroy those remaining few cells.

One interesting suggestion is to combine angiogenesis inhibitors with drugs which are made toxic by low oxygen levels (Harris, 1996). These drugs, as we have discussed in chapter 7, are harmless when they are surrounded by normal amounts of oxygen, but are turned into deadly poisons when the oxygen levels drop. With this drug combination, the angiogenesis inhibitors would destroy the blood vessels and drop the oxygen concentration inside the tumor, killing some cancer cells. Other cancer cells would probably be more resistant to the effects of low oxygen. As the blood vessels die, however, the lowered oxygen concentrations would activate the drug, which would then help to destroy the remaining cancer cells. This deadly combination might end up killing the tumor entirely, or it might leave a rim of living cells on the edge of the tumor, to be killed by conventional chemotherapy.

A paradox

Alert readers may have noticed one anomaly in some of the research we have discussed. Angiogenesis inhibitors prevent the growth of new blood vessels. Theoretically, they should not affect already formed ones. So they should be able to stop or slow growth of the tumor, but not shrink it. Yet, in some experiments, angiogenesis inhibitors actually shrink existing tumors (Barinaga, 1997a). How can this be? No one really knows the answer to this question (though researchers have undoubtedly been delighted with this pleasant surprise). One idea, however, is that the angiogenesis inhibitors shrink tumors because blood vessels are constantly being remodeled and the cells replaced (Barinaga, 1997a). If the inhibitors are present during this remodeling, then new parts of the blood vessel may be prevented from growing and replacing the bits that have died or been removed. Eventually, the whole vessel will disintegrate and be gone.

Blocking blood vessels with targeted blood clots

There is another way to block the cancer cells from getting blood, without stopping the formation of new blood vessels. This is to block existing blood vessels within the tumor. Of course, this treatment can be riskier than blocking angiogenesis. If blood vessels outside the tumor were blocked as well, the results could be disastrous. Heart attacks and strokes, for example, are the result of stopping blood flow to the heart or brain, respectively. Thorpe and colleagues have, however, come up with an interesting new way to block blood vessels in tumors, while leaving blood vessels in the rest of the body alone (Huang, 1997). They found a way to deliver a blood clotting protein called Tissue Factor specifically to tumor blood vessels. Tissue Factor is normally found outside all blood vessels. When a vessel is damaged, Tissue Factor slips inside, attaches to the endothelial cells and starts the blood clotting process. The researchers made a modified Tissue Factor which could be injected into the bloodstream, and does not attach anywhere except to the blood vessels inside tumors, where it triggers clot formation.

The details of this experiment are somewhat complex. First, they made genetically engineered cancer cells. These cells could trigger nearby blood vessels to make a protein called a MHC class II protein. Under ordinary conditions, endothelial cells do not make MHC II. The researchers injected the modified tumor cells into mice and allowed tumors to develop, complete with their MHC II carrying blood vessels. Then they modified Tissue Factor. They cut off the part which attaches it to endothelial cells, and gave it an artificial anchor which could only attach to MHC class II molecules. Essentially, they were making a Tissue Factor which could only trigger blood clotting when attached to MHC II. They injected this modified Tissue Factor into the blood of the mice with the tumors. The tissue factor attached to the tumor blood vessels and triggered blood clotting within minutes. Thirty eight percent of the tumors disappeared completely. In the others, the cells around the outside of the tumor survived (since they could getting nutrients and oxygen from blood vessels outside the tumor). The researchers suspect that these remaining cells could probably be killed by conventional chemotherapy.

This system is, of course, an artificial system. Human tumors are not genetically modified to bear molecules of our choice. Tissue Factor could, however, be modified to attach to other molecules as well. Researchers now need to find molecules which are found on tumor blood vessels but not on normal vessels. In fact, they believe that they have found some unique molecules on tumor blood vessels. A modified Tissue Factor directed against these molecules should be able to trigger clotting specifically in tumor blood vessels. The leader of this team estimates that this should be possible within a few years.

Destroying tumor blood vessels with guided chemotherapy

Other researchers are already using unique molecules on tumor blood vessels to guide toxic drugs to the tumor. Wadih Arap and colleagues have identified several molecules which seem to be found only on blood vessels inside some tumors (Arap, 1998). Arap's group has also made small pieces of protein which find and attach specifically to some of these molecules. When these protein pieces (called peptides) are linked to the cancer drug Doxorubicin, they can carry the drug directly to the tumor.

This has the advantage of concentrating the drug at the tumor site, and sparing normal cells from its toxicity. This peptide-linked Doxorubicin has been tested in mice with breast cancer. In this experiment, mice treated with ordinary Doxorubicin (not linked to the peptides) died either from the tumors or from drug poisoning (if very high doses were given). In contrast, mice given Doxorubicin attached to the targeting peptide had their tumors regress and lived much longer. The Doxorubicin seemed to work mainly by destroying blood vessels and cutting off the blood supply to the tumor (Barinaga, 1998a). It may also have spread into the tumor tissue itself and directly killed some cancer cells (Barinaga, 1998a). One nice thing about this treatment is that it can bypass the problem of drug resistance to Doxorubicin. Even if the tumor cells themselves mutate to make Doxorubicin less effective, normal endothelial cells do not mutate as readily (Barinaga, 1998a). They would be likely to remain sensitive to the drug, which would still be able to destroy the blood vessels. Another group of researchers has done a similar experiment, linking diphtheria toxin to the blood vessel growth factor VEGF (Barinaga, 1998). This modified toxin attaches to the VEGF receptor, abundant in new blood vessels such as are found in tumors. In their experiment, tumors in mice also regressed.

Looking outside the tumor - turning off the fibroblasts

Although targeting tumor blood vessels seems the obvious choice in attacking tumors through normal cells, there are a few other ideas as well. Some researchers, for example, think that tumor growth could be slowed by turning off cells called fibroblasts which surround the tumor. Fibroblasts are normal cells found everywhere in the body. They perform many important functions, including making some of the substances which bind together groups of cells and tissues, and participating in wound healing. Fibroblasts surrounding tumor cells, however, seem to be more active than fibroblasts in other tissues (Hall, 1995). They appear to have been stimulated by the cancer cells to produce growth factors and other proteins (Hall, 1995). There is a chance that, if these fibroblasts could be turned off, tumor growth and/or blood vessel growth might also be slowed. This idea is still in the early stages, although proteins identifying stimulated fibroblasts surrounding tumors have been identified (Hall, 1995).

Chapter 19

Phototherapy - using light to destroy cancer

One of the most surprising ways to destroy cancer cells uses a very simple ingredient - light. More than 90 years ago, a scientist discovered that single celled organisms treated with certain chemicals, then exposed to light, died (National Cancer Institute, 1998e). Neither the chemicals alone nor the light alone killed the cells (Figure 19.1). The chemicals, called photosensitizers, are harmless to cells by themselves; however, when they are stimulated by light, they become deadly. Based on this experience, researchers reasoned that the same combination of events might kill single cancer cells in the body - provided that a chemical could be chosen which was retained by cancer cells but not by normal cells. Such photosensitizers have since been found. This technique, called phototherapy, was first used in the 1970s to treat human skin tumors (van Hillegersberg, 1994) but has since been used for a wide variety of tumor types. It can be used either with the intention of curing the tumor or as a palliative treatment (therapy which decreases symptoms and increases the quality of life but is not expected to cure).

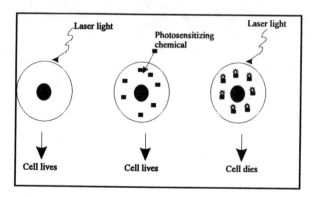

Figure 19.1. Neither laser light alone nor a photosensitizer alone are dangerous to cells, but when light activates the drug, it becomes deadly.

In phototherapy, a dose of a photosensitizing drug is injected into the blood. Afterward, the patient must wait for a time. During this waiting period, normal cells will first absorb the drug, then quickly eliminate it. Cancer cells, on the other hand, will retain the drug for longer. The waiting period can vary quite a bit between drugs; depending on the photosensitizer, it can last from hours to days (Dellian, 1996; Pharmacyclics, 1997). The patient's tumor is then exposed to light. In modern phototherapy, laser light is used. One advantage to laser light is that it is all a single wavelength (ordinary light is composed of many wavelengths) (National Cancer Institute, 1998b). Each photosensitizer responds best to a specific wavelength and the laser is matched to that wavelength. Laser light can also be focused onto the cancer, while ordinary light radiates in all directions. Laser light, therefore, also causes fewer side effects.

How phototherapy kills cells

Phototherapy kills cancer cells by generating free radicals inside the cell. Light stimulates the photosensitizing drug to expel an electron; this electron will then combine with oxygen to form a dangerous form of oxygen known as singlet oxygen (van Hillegersberg, 1994; Pharmacyclics, 1997). Single oxygen is a particularly effective free radical. It damages important molecules such as DNA and kills the cell (Figure 19.2). Phototherapy also seems to collapse the blood vessels in the tumor (remember that these are particularly fragile, disorganized blood vessels) (Boyle, 1996). This cuts off blood flow to the cancer cells and kills some of them.

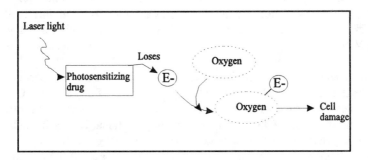

Figure 19.2.. Light stimulates a photosensitizing drug to expel an electron, which is picked up by oxygen to form a dangerous free radical.

There are also some hints that phototherapy may trigger the immune system to increase its activity against cancer cells. Scientists have noticed that, after phototherapy, immune cells called neutrophils and macrophages quickly enter the treated area (Krosl, 1995). Phototherapy also seems to make some of these macrophages more efficient at killing tumor cells. Some researchers speculate that this cell migration may be the beginning of an enhanced immune response against the tumor cells. One recent study combined phototherapy with treatments to stimulate the immune system, and dramatically increased the effectiveness of phototherapy (Korbelik, 1997). DBPMAF ("serum vitamin D3 binding protein derived macrophage activating factor") is a chemical from the blood which can stimulate macrophages. In this study, DBPMAF and phototherapy were used against squamous cell carcinomas, a type of skin cancer, in mice (Korbelik, 1997). DBPMAF alone had no effect on the tumors. Phototherapy alone cured 25 percent. When researchers added DBPMAF, however, all of the mice were cured.

Phototherapy appears to be a fairly safe treatment. The major side effect is skin sensitivity to light (National Cancer Institute, 1998e; Pharmacyclics, 1997). With some photosensitizers, this skin sensitivity may last six weeks or longer; unfortunately, sun screens are not completely effective in blocking the effect and patients must avoid sunlight for that time (National Cancer Institute, 1998e). Other side effects have been seen with some photosensitizers; these include nausea and vomiting, a metallic taste in the mouth, and sensitivity of the eyes to light (National Cancer Institute, 1998e). One study found an increased risk of developing some types of skin cancers after phototherapy. (Watson, 1997).

In general, phototherapy has been most effective against superficial tumors, tumors which are on a body surface and are fairly shallow. One reason is that the lasers used for most photosensitizers can only penetrate 1 centimeter below the surface of the body (National Cancer Institute, 1998b; National Cancer Institute, 1998e). Any part of the tumor below this limit will simply not be affected, regardless of how much photosensitizer it has accumulated. Another reason is that most of the current photosensitizers cannot be stimulated by wavelengths of light which can penetrate more deeply into the skin; even if the light could go deeper, it would do no good (Pharmacyclics, 1997). Recently, however, there has been an explosion of research into new photosensitizers and lasers which could expand these limits.

New photosensitizers and lasers

The effectiveness of phototherapy is determined mainly by two factors: the ability of the photosensitizer to concentrate in the cancer cells and the ability of the laser to reach and activate the photosensitizer (van Hillegersberg, 1994). The first photosensitizer used against cancer was a crude mixture of chemicals from the blood called porphyrins (van Hillegersberg, 1994). Newer photosensitizers, such as porfimer sodium, are considerably more purified (van Hillegersberg, 1994). A new chemical called Photofrin (dihematoporphyrin ether/ester, DHE) has recently been approved by the FDA for clinical trials (National Cancer Institute, 1998e).

Cancer researchers are working to develop other photosensitizers which concentrate more quickly in the tumor, have reduced side effects, and are more effective. A dozen or more new photosensitizers are being tested, including chemicals such as the porphycenes, Texaphyrin, benzoporpyrin, 5-aminolevulinic acid and Hypericin (van Hillegersberg, 1994; VanderWerf, 1996; Tong, 1996).

One recent study, for example, tested chemicals called porphycenes, which scientists hoped would be concentrated in the tumor cells more quickly than the current photosensitizers. In this study, hamsters with melanomas were given either porphycenes or Photofrin, then treated with laser light (Dellian, 1996). The hamsters achieved complete remission with either treatment. There was, however, a significant advantage to using the porphycenes, particularly one called CBPn. Hamsters receiving CBPn could be treated with the laser five minutes after receiving the drug, compared to 24 hours for Photofrin. This could be a significant advantage to a human patient. Instead of prolonged waits, which can last for days, patients could be able to complete a course of phototherapy in a single outpatient visit. A second advantage to porphycenes was that six-fold lower doses could be given, compared to Photofrin; with lower doses, fewer side effects should be seen. Other photosensitizers have also shown promise in the laboratory. For example, Hypericin (VanderWerf, 1996), and a group of carbacyanine dyes (Lipshutz, 1994) have been able to kill a variety of cancer cells grown in the laboratory, with minimal damage to normal body cells. The newest photosensitizers in the news are, however, the Texaphyrins.

Texaphyrin - a "Texas sized" photosensitizer

Texaphyrins are those big "Texas sized" porphyrins, attached to various metals, mentioned previously as radiation sensitizers. Texaphyrins are turning out to be quite promising in phototherapy as well. Lutetium Texaphyrin (Lu-Tex) has been used as a photosensitizer for a variety of skin cancers (Yuen, 1997). Lu-Tex has several advantages over other photosensitizers. It rapidly leaves normal cells, including normal skin cells (Pharmacyclics, 1997). This greatly reduces skin sensitivity to light. Lu-Tex can also be used much more quickly than most photosensitizers. Light treatment can start as soon as three hours after the drug is given (Pharmacyclics, 1997).

Lu-Tex shares these advantages, of course, with the porphycenes. One unique property of Lu-Tex, however, is that it responds to wavelengths of light which penetrate more deeply into the body than is usual in phototherapy (Pharmacyclics, 1997).This allows Lu-Tex to be used in somewhat deeper tumors and also in melanomas, which can have a pigment which blocks light. Most other photosensitizers respond to wavelengths that can penetrate very shallowly, and can be used only on tumors that are 1 to 3 millimeters thick. Lu-Tex has been used on 2-4 mm tumors in mice with an 86 percent cure rate (Pharmacyclics, 1997). Even tumors which were 3 to 7 mm responded to some extent. The improved light penetration also allows phototherapy to be used in skin cancer patients with darker skin, in which pigments block light; previously, phototherapy was limited to patients with light skin.

Lutetium Texaphyrin is in the early stages of cancer trials in humans. Some of the early research was reported at the 1997 American Society of Clinical Oncology meeting (Yuen, 1997). In one study, 35 patients with skin cancers (which had metastasized to the skin from other sites) were given a single dose of lutetium Texaphyrin, then treated with laser light 3 to 8 hours later (Yuen, 1997). Of 104 cancer sites on these patients, 26% regressed completely, and 18 percent regressed partially. The side effects were not severe in most patients, and five of six patients who had a second dose of Lu-Tex had an improved response after the second dose.

Further trials are expected soon. Gadolinium Texaphyrin is also being investigated for use in phototherapy (Pharmacyclics, 1997). One advantage to gadolinium Texaphyrin is that it can be detected by MRI (magnetic resonance imaging), and so its exact location can be determined before starting laser treatment.

Clinical trials of phototherapy

Phototherapy is not useful for all cancers. It cannot be used for large tumors, since light cannot penetrate far into tissues. Phototherapy also needs oxygen to be effective (van Hillegersberg, 1994); therefore, it is not likely to be useful in the poorly-oxygenated centers of larger tumors, even if light could penetrate that far. Phototherapy has, however, been successfully used in a number of small surface cancers, particularly skin cancers (National Cancer Institute, 1998b). It is usually expected to be most effective in early cancers (Evensen, 1995), although it sometimes has been of benefit even at later stages (Tong, 1996).

Phototherapy has been particularly useful for a skin cancer called mycosis fungoides (Watson, 1997). Although "mycosis fungoides" might sound like a fungus infection, it is actually a form of white blood cell cancer in which the cancer cells are found mainly in the skin. There are several options for treating mycosis fungoides. One effective treatment is external radiation combined with a type of chemotherapy where DNA alkylating drugs are applied to the skin (Berkow, 1992). This treatment can, however, have considerable side effects. This can be an important consideration in this disease, where most patients are over 50, and can expect to live for 7 to 10 years with the disease, even without treatment (Berkow, 1992). Phototherapy is, however, an effective and less toxic alternative. In early cases of mycosis fungoides, phototherapy seems to be effective alone (Watson, 1997). It has also been helpful in advanced mycosis fungoides, in combination with other treatments (such as the cytokine interferon gamma) (Watson, 1997; Tong, 1996). In one study, for example, 36 of 39 patients with advanced mycosis fungoides responded to treatment with phototherapy and interferon gamma (Kuzel, 1995). Most of these patients (62% of the 36) had a complete response, while 28% had at least a partial response. Twenty nine of the patients were still alive at the time the study was reported (5 years after the first patient had been treated).

Phototherapy has also been useful for small tumors which are deeper in the body. One way to get light to tumors which are deep in the body (but which are still on the surface of some organ or otherwise accessible) is to use fiber optics (National Cancer Institute, 1998b; van Hillegersberg, 1994). Fiber optic cables are essentially tubes which can direct laser light into the body. They are maneuvered through openings (either surgical or natural) until they reach the site of the cancer; laser light is then directed down the cable and shines out the end (Figure 19.3). Since the 1980s, phototherapy has been used to treat tumors inside the lungs' air passages (Sutedja, 1996). When these tumors become large enough, they can block air flow. Treating a large airway tumor with phototherapy is not likely to cure it, but it will decrease its size and allow the patient to breathe more comfortably (Sutedja, 1996). More recently, phototherapy has been used in attempts to cure early lung cancers, as well as cancers of the bladder, esophagus, brain, and ovaries (Kato, 1996; National Cancer Institute, 1998b). In a (phase II) clinical study using phototherapy to treat early stages of lung, esophageal, stomach, cervical, and bladder cancers (from 1989-1992), the treatment appears to have been successful in at least half of those cases (Kato, 1996).

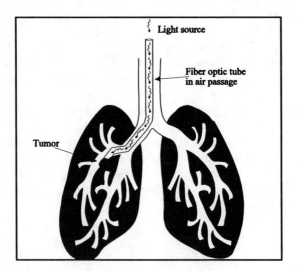

Figure 19.3. Tumors deep inside the lung's airways can be treated by phototherapy, with light directed down a fiber optic cable.

Phototherapy can occasionally help patients with tumors which are resistant to other forms of treatment. Nasopharyngeal carcinoma, for example, is a cancer located in the nose and throat. It can be treated with radiation; however, in cases where the cancer returns after radiation treatment, there is no effective treatment (Tong, 1996). In one study, twelve patients with such tumors were treated with phototherapy as a last-ditch effort to treat the returned tumors (Tong, 1996). Eight patients were treated with the intention of curing the cancer. Three of the eight patients had no signs of cancer nine to twelve months after phototherapy. Four patients had tumors with no potential for a cure; they were treated with the intention only of decreasing the size of the tumor. For three of these four patients, phototherapy improved their quality of life.

Combination therapies

Like many cancer treatments, phototherapy may be most effective when it is used in combination with other forms of therapy. Researchers are studying combinations of phototherapy with hyperthermia, chemotherapy, radiation, and surgery (van Hillegersberg, 1994). Phototherapy may be particularly useful in destroying residual cancer cells after surgery; light could simply be shined into the surgical area before closing the site. An intriguing idea is to use phototherapy to remove cancer cells from blood or bone marrow stem cells during high dose chemotherapy with autologous stem cell transplant. In one study, several photosensitizing drugs were effective in destroying cancerous white blood cells without destroying normal blood cell stem cells (Gulati, 1994). This treatment took an hour, and seems to be quite practical. It could be very useful in increasing the success rate of high dose chemotherapy.

Chapter 20

Hyperthermia -turning up the heat

Hyperthermia is a unique way of killing cancer cells: with a fever. Some readers may have heard of hyperthermia as something to avoid, a life threatening condition on hot days when an active body overheats. But controlled hyperthermia is also a promising form of treatment for cancer. It was born in the 1970's, when researchers noticed that some cancer patients went into remission when their internal body temperatures were raised (Pontiggia, 1996). They discovered that when the body temperature of a human, ordinarily at 37°C, is raised to 42°C, the increased temperatures kill some tumor cells (but spare normal cells) (Pontiggia, 1996). In a sense, hyperthermia is an artificial fever, targeted specifically at cancer cells.

There are now several different forms of hyperthermia: whole body, regional, and local. Whole body hyperthermia is the heating of a patient's entire body, used in cases where the cancer has spread throughout the body. Warm water blankets, warm wax, high temperature chambers, or thermal coils (like those in electric blankets) are used (National Cancer Institute, 1997a). Regional hyperthermia is heat applied to a small part of the body, perhaps an arm or a leg. Magnets or high energy devices are placed over the area to heat that segment of the body (National Cancer Institute, 1997a). An alternative is to warm the blood supplying that area of the body. In local hyperthermia, heat is applied directly to the tumor itself, sparing the patient some discomfort. High frequency sound waves or lasers or microwaves are sometimes used to heat the tumor in local hyperthermia (National Cancer Institute, 1997a). Another possibility is to insert wires into the tumor to conduct heat, or tubes carrying warm water (National Cancer Institute, 1997a).

How hyperthermia kills cancer cells

Researchers are still figuring out how hyperthermia actually destroys tumors - and why it affects cancer cells more than normal cells. Heat can kill a cell in more than one way. Very high temperatures will, of course, destroy any cell, as anyone who has ever burned himself on a hot stove can testify. This destruction essentially bursts apart the cell (biologists call the process "necrosis") and may cook the proteins inside. The temperatures usually used in normal hyperthermia are not high enough to destroy cells in this way. In fact, if they did, then normal cells might be expected to die in equal numbers to cancer cells. Instead, many researchers believe that hyperthermia triggers the cancer cell's innate program for cell suicide (also called apoptosis) (Shchepotin, 1997). Essentially, hyperthermia may send a death signal to the cell, to which the cell meekly responds!

Hyperthermia can also destroy tumor cells in other ways. For instance, it may stimulate the immune system to attack the tumor by increasing its visibility to the immune cells. Hyperthermia can increase the amount of some proteins on the surfaces of cancer cells (Takahashi, 1995). These proteins are like red flags, identifying the cancer cell to the body as "not self," or something that doesn't belong in the body and should be destroyed. Increasing these proteins may, therefore, help the immune system to recognize and attack the tumor. There is also some evidence that hyperthermia directly stimulates some immune cells (called macrophages) to kill cancer cells (Pontiggia, 1996).

Hyperthermia also seems to contribute to cell death by decreasing blood flow in the tumor (Engin, 1994a; Engin, 1994b). It appears to collapse the fragile, poorly formed blood vessels within the tumor, at temperatures where normal blood vessels are not affected. One effect is, of course, to starve the cancer cells of necessary nutrients and oxygen. Another effect may be to further increase the temperature inside the tumor, heating it more than surrounding normal tissues (Engin, 1994a; Engin, 1994b); this may aid in damaging cancer cells without harming normal cells.

The major side effects of hyperthermia seem to be general discomfort and sometimes pain in the area being treated (Gonzalez Gonzalez, 1995; Pontiggia, 1995). This discomfort may be enough to halt treatments; nearly a fifth (17 percent) of the treatments in one study were prematurely stopped due to pain and discomfort (Gonzalez Gonzalez, 1995).

Clinical studies of hyperthermia

Hyperthermia has been promising for the treatment of head and neck tumors, breast cancer, and melanomas (Engin, 1994a). In many cases, hyperthermia has also been used to increase the effectiveness of treatments such as radiation or chemotherapy. It may do this in a variety of ways. For example, it may inhibit the repair of DNA damage (Engin, 1994a). After radiation therapy or chemotherapy, cancer cells can sometimes repair their DNA damage, recover, and survive. When hyperthermia is added to these treatments, repair may be inhibited and more cancer cells are killed.

Hyperthermia seems to be particularly useful when it is combined with radiation. For example, some patients with tumors on body surfaces may respond better to radiation and hyperthermia than to radiotherapy alone (Engin, 1994b;). This combination was also useful, in several clinical trials, in patients with breast cancers that had returned after conventional treatment (Vernon, 1996). In these studies, hyperthermia may have helped to produce tumor regression in patients who could not tolerate high doses of radiation. Radiation and hyperthermia may turn out to be effective in colon cancer, as well (Gonzalez Gonzalez, 1995). In one study, 72 colon cancer patients were treated with regional hyperthermia combined with radiotherapy. Of these patients, 15 percent went into remission after treatment, 17% survived for 3 years, and 75 percent at least had a decrease in their symptoms. Although these results are less than spectacular, the researchers noted that the actual temperatures inside these internal tumors did not reach the target of 41 °C (the average temperature was around 40 °C). More effective heating of the cancer itself, they concluded, might produce better results.

Hyperthermia and chemotherapy may also be a useful combination. Hyperthermia seems to increase the sensitivity of cancer cells to many drugs, and may even convert some otherwise non-toxic drugs into very toxic ones (Engin, 1994b). Hyperthermia seems to be particularly effective in combination with the drugs called alkylating agents and with cis-platinum (Engin, 1994b). Whole body hyperthermia, combined with the drug melphalan, may be promising for deadly cancers of the pancreas and malignant melanoma (Robins, 1997), and for colon cancers in mice (Shchepotin, 1997). Hyperthermia may even have benefits in patients with metastatic breast cancer, a cancer which has a particularly dismal record for treatment (Pontiggia, 1995). In one study, 59 patients with metastatic breast cancer were treated with hyperthermia, low doses of chemotherapy drugs and treatments which manipulated the immune system (Pontiggia, 1995). These patients had cancers which did not respond to conventional treatment and they were expected to survive an average of 8 to 9 months. With this combination therapy, however, a significant number seemed to beat the odds. Twenty three patients went into complete remission and, of these, 14 were still alive 17 to 80 months later. The other nine patients had 20 to 40 months of life without disease symptoms before the cancer returned. It is difficult, of course, to dissect each part of this treatment to determine what role it played; nevertheless, the researchers believed that hyperthermia made a significant contribution to the effectiveness of the therapy.

Hyperthermia is still, however, a relatively new treatment. Its advantages are that it is simple and fairly nontoxic, and seems to be reasonably effective in enhancing other therapies. In addition, it is not affected by oxygen levels in a tumor (Engin, 1994b); this may make it a useful combination with treatments that can only kill well-oxygenated cells. At one time, physicians always tried to suppress fevers, thinking that they damaged the body. These days, biologists have learned that a fever is often useful (as long as it not too high) in helping the immune system kill invading microorganisms. It seems rather ironic that a simple fever may also turn out to be useful in combating such a deadly and complex disease as cancer.

Chapter 21

Apoptosis - asking the cancer cells to kill themselves

All normal cells have "death pathways" inside the cell; when these pathways are triggered, they kill the cell. Cancer researchers have recently become very interested in this process, called apoptosis or cell suicide. One reason for this sudden popularity is the startling news that many cancer treatments actually work by turning on apoptosis (Hannun, 1997). Radiation, hyperthermia, and the retinoids can all turn on cell suicide pathways. Hormone withdrawal in hormone-dependent tumors (such as anti-androgens for prostate cancers) may also cause death by apoptosis. Many chemotherapy drugs seem to stimulate apoptosis. Tumor cells which are unable to commit suicide may, in fact, be resistant to many cancer treatments (Hannun, 1997). Apoptosis is, therefore, becoming very important to cancer treatment. If apoptosis can be understood, some researchers hope that resistant cancer cells might be made more susceptible to treatment. Some even hope that they might be able to bypass the conventional drugs altogether and directly turn on the death signals inside a cancer cell.

How a cell dies - two types of cell death

The are two basic ways that a cell can die, called necrosis and apoptosis. Necrosis is a messy bursting open of the cell, with the contents spread everywhere, and immune cells coming in to clean up the debris. The immune system responds to necrosis with inflammation, a process that results in the physical symptoms of redness, swelling, warmth and pain. It's the same response you get when you hit your thumb with a hammer or have an infected cut. Necrosis usually results from outside factors that damage cells: viruses bursting open the cell, bacterial poisons destroying the cell, or physical damage.

Apoptosis, on the other hand, is a cell that simply kills itself. For this reason, it is often called cell suicide. Apoptosis is a "death pathway" found in all cells. All it requires is the right trigger to set it off. When it is triggered, the cell quietly cuts up its DNA, kills itself, and breaks up into neat membrane enclosed packages ready for pickup by the nearest scavenging immune cell. No inflammation results and the body barely notices that anything has happened. Apoptosis is an important part of development in the embryo, when cells die to form organs. For example, when the cells between the fingers die, four fingers and a thumb are made from what was a shapeless mitt before. Apoptosis is also important during the rest of an organism's life, as cells grow old and must die, or surplus or mutated cells must be killed (Nagata, 1997). In the immune system, for example, short lived cells called neutrophils are produced in tremendous numbers every day. Unless an infection is present, they are unneeded. Most of the time, therefore, tremendous numbers of neutrophils must also die every day. If this death occurred by necrosis, it would be an uncomfortable and even dangerous mess of constant inflammation; by apoptosis, it is barely noticeable.

How apoptosis works

Researchers are just beginning to understand the triggers that initiate apoptosis, the pathways that deliver that signal to the nucleus, and the final destructive responses inside the cell.

The triggers

The first component of apoptosis is the signal received by the cancer cell, which triggers the apoptosis pathway. There is more than one signal to trigger apoptosis.

Some apoptosis signals come from outside the cell. Cells actually carry "death receptors" on their surfaces to receive these signals. The signal itself is usually a molecule from another cell that attaches to this receptor. One of the better known signals is the Fas-L molecule, which attaches to a Fas molecule on the recipient cell (Figure 21.1). For example, some cells of the immune system kill their targets by simply linking FasL on their surfaces to Fas on the target cell (Nagata, 1997); in effect, they politely ask the target to kill itself and it obliges! Tumor necrosis factor (TNF), a protein made by the immune system, can trigger apoptosis by attaching to the tumor necrosis factor receptor (Hannun, 1997; Barinaga, 1996a; Nagata, 1997). A third suicide signal, called TRAIL ("TNF-related apoptosis inducing factor"), also comes from outside the cell (Gura, 1997b; Nagata, 1997). Several other new external apoptosis triggers have also recently been discovered, although little is known about them yet (Nagata, 1997).

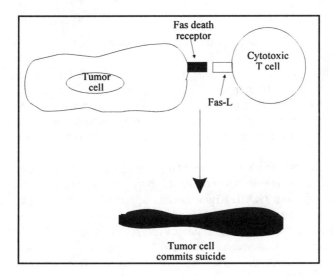

Figure 21.1 Some immune cells can kill cancer cells by triggering the Fas death receptor.

There are signals which come from inside a cell, as well. For example, damage inside the cell can trigger apoptosis by turning on p53. P53 is the checkpoint molecule which stops the cell cycle when DNA is damaged. The p53 protein seems to do more, however, than simply check for mutations. It also detects a number of other abnormalities inside the cell. For example, having too few building blocks for DNA synthesis can turn on p53 (Levine, 1997). So can low oxygen levels (Levine, 1997). Some researchers speculate that p53 might act like an internal coordinator for the cell, to assess damage from a variety of sources and organize a response. It might even be able to kill some cancer cells when they begin to grow quickly and their local supply of oxygen drops (Levine, 1997)

Mutations in trigger molecules in cancer cells

It should not be too surprising that many cancer cells have mutations in apoptosis triggering molecules. The *p53* genes, for example, have been mutated in slightly more than half of all human cancers (Levine, 1997). This mutation can prevent cancer cells from detecting DNA damage and committing suicide after many different cancer treatments.

The external death signal TRAIL is interesting to cancer researchers because cancer cells may actually be more susceptible than healthy cells to signals from TRAIL (Gura, 1997b). Apparently, normal cells have two receptors for the TRAIL molecule (Figure 21.2): one sends the death signal, but the other one is a dummy receptor, that attaches to TRAIL but sends no signals anywhere (Gura, 1997b). When TRAIL reaches a normal cell, it attaches to the dummy receptors, and is, therefore, harmless. Oddly enough, cancer cells tend to have only the real TRAIL receptor, which sends the suicide signal right into the cell. (No one knows why cancer cells are missing the other receptor). Genentech company (S. San Francisco) and Immunex Corporation (Seattle) are testing the TRAIL protein in rodents with cancer (Gura, 1997b). Theoretically, this normal body protein should be able to trigger apoptosis in cancer cells, but be ignored by normal cells.

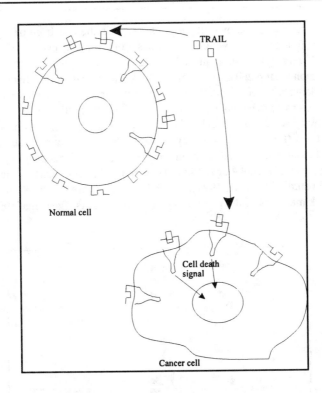

Figure 21.2. Cancer cells lack the "dummy receptor" which can protect normal cells from the death signal sent by TRAIL.

The pathways to death

Although there are many potential triggers for apoptosis (Figure 21.3), the messages from all of these triggering molecules are eventually sent to a final "death program," which triggers cell death. At its beginning, however, the pathway from each trigger may be different. Some death signals, such as Fas, seem to lead directly to the death program (Barinaga, 1996a). Others, such as TNF receptor or p53, seem to choose from either pathways leading to cell death or "rescue" pathways which prevent the death signal from continuing (Barinaga, 1996a; Levine, 1997).

Perhaps the best known of these pathways is the one from p53. It is a branching pathway, which sometimes stops the cell cycle and allows DNA repair, and sometimes leads to cell death (Levine, 1997). The decision to stop cell division gives DNA repair systems the chance to fix the damage before the cell passes on mutations. If, however, damage is too extensive to be repaired, apoptosis is the only solution. The part of the pathway which blocks cell division requires the cooperation of several proteins (Levine, 1997). If any of these proteins are abnormal, the cell cycle may not stop. At least one of the members of this pathway - p53, p16, cyclin D1, cdk4 or RB - has been mutated in most cancers that have been studied (Levine, 1997). Several new drugs are being developed to block members of the p53 pathways in cancer cells (Barinaga, 1997b).

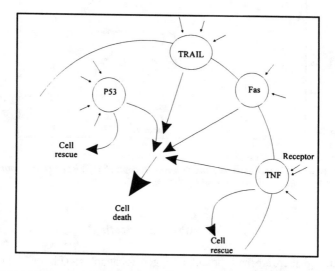

Figure 21.3. Signals from a variety of death receptors can lead to apoptosis. Sometimes, the cell can be saved from death by rescue pathways.

Proteins which influence a cell's susceptibility to death

The cells's decision to commit suicide is not taken lightly by the body. For example, in the p53 pathway, signals from growth factors can sometimes block apoptosis (Levine, 1997). A number of other factors seem to influence the decision, as well. There are even molecules in the cell whose jobs are to help decide whether to commit to apoptosis or not. Among them are the Bcl-2 family proteins, and NF-κB.

A large group ("family") of proteins - including members Bcl-2, Bax, Bcl-x, Bad, Bag, Bak and Bik - seems to have the job of deciding how susceptible a cell will be to apoptosis (Hannun, 1997; Nagata, 1997). Some, such as Bcl-2, Bcl-xL, Bcl-w, and Mcl-1 tend to turn off apoptosis; others, such as Bax, Bik, Bad and Bcl-xs tend to promote apoptosis (Hannun, 1997; Nagata, 1997). Some researchers think that this group of proteins, as a whole, controls the cell's current susceptibility to apoptosis (Nagata, 1997). For example, if a cell were to have a lot of Bax and Bik, but very little Bcl-2, it would commit suicide relatively easily. A lot of Bcl-2 and little Bax, and apoptosis would become more difficult to carry out. In fact, the *bcl-2* gene is overactive in approximately half of all human cancers (Barinaga, 1997b). These cancers can be tough to kill. Excess Bcl-2, for example, is associated with a poor response to chemotherapy (Hannun, 1997).

Drugs which may be able to inhibit Bcl-2 are being tested in animals, and some human clinical trials have begun or will soon begin (Barinaga, 1997b). In one preliminary study in humans, one of nine patients with advanced lymphoma had a complete remission when treated with Bcl-2 inhibitors, and another patient had a partial remission (Barinaga, 1997b)

Another protein, NF-κB, has many roles in the cell. One of them seems to be rescuing the cell from death (Barinaga, 1996b). Unfortunately, some drugs and radiation may be able to turn on NF-κB (Barinaga, 1996b). In a sense, these agents are a bit ambivalent. On the one hand, they turn on a pathway to cell death. On the other, they turn on a protein which can stop cell death. Some researchers hope to improve cancer treatment by combining radiation or chemotherapy with drugs that turn off NF-κB. In early experiments, blocking NF-κB could, in fact, improve cancer cell killing by chemotherapy (Barinaga, 1996b).

The end of the story -
the final common pathway to cell death

Once the cell has made a decision to actually commit to apoptosis, it apparently triggers a final death program, which actually kills the cell. A group of proteins called the caspases seem to actually carry out apoptosis, apparently by chewing apart important molecules in the cell (Barinaga, 1996a; Nagata, 1997). The caspases are absolutely required for apoptosis to occur, but other proteins seem to be involved as well. Very little is known about these last stages (Nagata, 1997).

A Summary - how such different treatments as chemotherapy,
radiation and retinoids can all turn on apoptosis

Drugs and radiation which damage DNA. Drugs which damage microtubules. Low oxygen levels. Withdrawal of growth factors. How can so many different treatments all trigger apoptosis? Y. A. Hannun (1997) has proposed an explanation. First, he suggests, chemotherapy, radiation, and other treatments destroy their specific targets in the cell. For example, alkylating drugs damage DNA and drugs which affect microtubules injure the cell skeleton. At this point, the cell damage is evaluated by the cell, through a variety of pathways which decide whether repair is possible or whether the cell should instead commit to apoptosis. DNA damage, for example, would be assessed through p53. Other pathways would evaluate other types of damage. The chemotherapy drug Doxorubicin, for example, seems to increase Fas-L on the cell surface of leukemic cells, making suicide more likely (Hannun, 1997). If the cell determined that the damage was extensive enough, then the signals from these different sources would feed into the final common pathway, where caspases actually carry out cell death.

The implications of all of this: how to ask a cell to kill itself

The ultimate goal of apoptosis research is, of course, to find better ways to kill cancer cells. One suggestion is to screen cancer cells for defective genes in the apoptosis pathways, then treat them to reverse the defect (Hannun, 1997; Barinaga, 1997b). For instance, cells missing p53 could have that gene transferred into the cell before chemotherapy with drugs that damage DNA. Cells which have excess Bcl-2 might be treated to suppress Bcl-2 production before treating the cancer with conventional therapy (Hannun, 1997). In fact, there is already evidence that blocking Bcl-2 in some resistant leukemia cells can make them susceptible to apoptosis (Hannun, 1997).

Another way to kill resistant cancer cells would be to simply ignore treatments that trigger mutated pathways and choose a treatment that acts on an intact apoptosis pathway (Hannun, 1997). For example, in cells resistant to chemotherapy due to defective p53, Fas-L (specifically aimed at cancer cells) or the TRAIL protein might work. Alternatively, a drug could be chosen which triggers a pathway which doesn't involve p53. Some researchers even suggest bypassing the early stages of apoptosis altogether and directly triggering a later step (Hannun, 1997). For example, some prostate cancer cells are thought to have defects in the apoptosis pathway. These cells continue to grow after suppression of androgens in the body. They seem to be able to perform the final steps of apoptosis, but are apparently missing something needed for the first step (Furuya, 1994). One way to get them to commit suicide is to bypass that step with the drug Thapsigargin, which triggers apoptosis by raising calcium levels (Furuya, 1994). Direct triggering of the caspases has also been suggested. As Y.A. Hannun (1997) points out, however, this would require "significantly more" understanding of apoptosis pathways, particularly of the final steps. Accidentally triggering caspases in all cells of the body would have rather drastic effects!

Finally, there is a particularly clever approach, which is to actually exploit the cancer cell's defect to kill it. One new cancer treatment, in fact, does just this. In this treatment, a virus has been modified to only kill cells which lack p53 - in other words, cancer cells (Hannun, 1997; Barinaga, 1997b). Researchers made the virus by modifying an adenovirus (a human cold virus) which can't infect cells unless it disables p53. The normal adenovirus carries proteins to disable p53. Researchers simply took out these proteins to create the cancer-killing virus. Since this modified virus cannot disable p53, it can only infect cells which already have p53 disabled (Barinaga, 1997b). In a healthy body, with a cancer lacking p53, this means that the virus can specifically kill the cancer cells, without bothering the normal ones. This virus has already been promising in human clinical trials. In early trials, it had no serious side effects in 32 patients with head and neck tumors (Barinaga, 1997b). In 12 of these patients, the tumors shrank up to 90 percent.

Unfortunately, this technique is not yet useful for metastatic cancer, and would be awkward to use for deeper tumors: the virus must be injected directly into the tumors (Barinaga, 1997b). With technical advances, however, this virus might turn out to be very useful in the many human cancers which are missing p53.

Chapter 22

The immune system

The immune system is a remarkable group of organs and cells which defend the body against invaders of every sort. The immune system has a formidable task: it must size up an invader, decide how to best respond to it, and coordinate a rapid, effective response - before the invader has a chance to do much damage. This remarkable feat is performed by immune cells, also known as white blood cells. These cells are made by the bone marrow, the tissue in the center of the bones. There are quite a few different types of white blood cells, and each has a specific role to play in the immune response. Immune cells do not function autonomously; they all interact with each other in an ever-changing ballet of cells. Each cell, however, has a specific part to play.

The cells of the immune system

There are basically two different types of cells in the immune system. One set, often referred to as "innate immunity," acts as the first line of defense against invaders. These cells include neutrophils, eosinophils, and basophils (collectively called the granulocytes), macrophages and Natural Killer cells. These cells are ready to respond to an invader the moment it enters the body. Each of them has a specialized function to perform. Natural Killer cells kill any body cells which have been infected by a virus. They also destroy cancer cells. Eosinophils and basophils help to eliminate parasites. Neutrophils kill bacteria. Macrophages are perhaps the most versatile of these cells: they destroy bacteria, kill cancer cells, participate in the healing of wounds, and have other functions, as well. Although this group of cells might sound impressive, it has some limitations. For instance, these cells are not able to respond differently to different types of threats - or, even, sometimes, to recognize a threat. A macrophage, for example, simply destroys anything in its path which is small enough to take inside the cell; it doesn't matter whether it is a bacterium, a bunch of cell debris, or just a globule of fat. These cells also cannot, by themselves, escalate their responses in response to an increasing threat. Finally, they carry no memory of invaders. If these cells were the only participants in the immune system, the body would have to endure repeated attacks from the same organism, with no better response the 30th time than the first. A person suffering from a bout of measles, for example, could look forward to getting measles again and again.

A person who gets measles, however, does not usually get measles again. This is due to the second type of cells in an immune response, the B and T lymphocytes. B and T cells can escalate their responses each time an invader is met; after the first encounter, they may respond so efficiently that they completely prevent any future attacks by that same organism. They can also distinguish between different types of threats, and respond differently to each. Not only can they tell a virus from a bacterium, but they can even detect the differences between two types of viruses or two different cells. Finally, they can produce proteins which stimulate the cells involved in innate immunity, making them more effective and better able to respond to threats.

T and B lymphocytes

T and B lymphocytes come from the bone marrow, like the other immune cells, but they get some special education after they are released. T lymphocytes finish their development in the thymus, an organ in the chest. Here, each T cell develops the ability to respond to a tiny piece of a single protein, called an antigen. (Anything the immune system responds to is called an antigen.) Each T cell can only respond to one antigen and to no others. As a consequence of this, the body must make massive numbers of T cells, to recognize all of the potential invaders it could encounter. T cells also learn to distinguish antigens which belong in the body, or "self," from antigens which do not. Actually, this is done in a simple, rather brutal way. Those T cells which would react against antigens that are normally found in the body are destroyed; only the T lymphocytes which do not recognize "self" are allowed to mature. One group of T cells, called helper T cells, becomes specialized to aid other cells of the immune system, particularly other lymphocytes. Another group of T cells, the cytotoxic T cells, specializes in killing body cells which have been invaded by a virus or which have become cancer cells.

B cells also continue to develop after they leave the bone marrow. Like T cells, B cells respond to only one antigen each. B cells which recognize self antigens may also be destroyed, although they seem to be controlled less strictly than T cells. The purpose of B cells is to make antibodies.

Cell Type	Functions
LYMPHOCYTES	
Helper T cells	Aid other cells by secreting cytokines; necessary for cytotoxic T cells and B cells to respond effectively
Cytotoxic T cells	Kill cells which have been infected by a virus and tumor cells; require helper T cell help
Natural Killer cells	Kill cells which have been infected by a virus and tumor cells; do not require helper T cell help
B cells	Produce antibodies; generally require helper T cell help
ANTIGEN PRESENTING CELLS	
Macrophages	Destroy bacteria and cancer cells, clean up cell debris, display antigens to helper T cells
Dendritic cells	Display antigens to helper T cells
GRANULOCYTES	
Neutrophils	Eat and destroy bacteria, clean up cell debris, may kill cancer cells

Interactions of B cells, T cells and antigen presenting cells: the immune response

The bone marrow makes tremendous numbers of lymphocytes, but it must respond to many different antigens; therefore, it only makes a few lymphocytes to recognize any single invader. This small number of cells must be expanded by an immune response before there will be enough cells to deal with any invasion. Normally, lymphocytes are also in a resting state; they must be "turned on" before they can defend the body against invaders. In fact, an immune response is designed to do only two basic things: increase the number of lymphocytes available to deal with that antigen, and turn them on. These activities usually occur in small organs called the lymph nodes or in an abdominal organ called the spleen.

Lymph nodes are found in strategic locations throughout the body, along a network of small tubes called lymphatic vessels. The lymphatic vessels return a fluid called lymph from the tissues to the blood. As the lymph percolates back to the blood, the lymph nodes sit along the lymphatic vessels and collect antigens carried in the lymph; the lymph nodes essentially monitor whether any infection or abnormality is occurring "upstream" of them. These collected antigens are constantly displayed to all of the B and T lymphocytes in the body. Large collections of lymphocytes are found in lymph nodes, but the cells don't just sit in a node and wait for antigens to come to them. Instead, they travel constantly throughout the body, patrolling for invaders. They enter lymph nodes from the blood or lymphatic vessels, percolate slowly through the lymph nodes, then continue their travels throughout the body. In this way, each lymphocyte monitors all of the lymph nodes in the body to see if its antigen can be found anywhere. When lymphocytes encounter something that should not be in the body, such as a piece of a virus, a bacterium, or a cancer cell, they pause in a local lymph node, interact with each other, and generate an immune response to deal with the threat.

Alerting the helper T cells

The central cell in any immune response is the helper T cell. These cells must coordinate the responses of all of the other cells in the immune system; without them, B cells and cytotoxic T cells are essentially paralyzed. The first step in an immune response is, therefore, to turn on the helper T cells. Nature has designed a complicated system to turn T cells on. (These complications probably help to keep the immune system from being turned on accidentally). Helper T cells require several different stimuli before they become active. The most important requirement is that they must find their antigen; in this way, resources are not wasted on useless T cells during an immune response. Helper T cells cannot, however, recognize antigens which are simply floating by in their surroundings. They must have their antigen shown to them in a sort of display case, called an MHC II molecule, on another cell (Figure 22.1). This is the job of the antigen presenting cells.

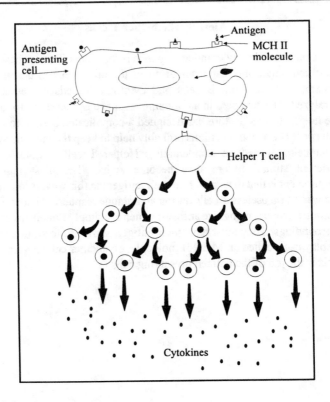

Figure 22.1. Antigen presenting cells show antigens to helper T cells and stimulate them to divide and produce cytokines.

The two major types of antigen presenting cells are the macrophages and dendritic cells (and B cells, in some situations that we won't concern ourselves with). Dendritic cells are probably the more important of the two. Dendritic cells are like a surveillance system which constantly picks up antigens and shows helper T cells what antigens are present in the body. Dendritic cells are found throughout the body. They collect proteins in their surroundings and display pieces of them in MHC II molecules. Most of the time, dendritic cells simply display bits of proteins from normal body cells. When the body is infected, however, they pick up pieces of the invader and display some of them as well. Dendritic cells periodically travel to the nearest lymph nodes, carrying their burden of antigens; in fact, most antigens probably reach lymph nodes already displayed on dendritic cells. If a passing helper T cell sees its antigen on a dendritic cell in a lymph node, it comes to a stop, settles down and responds to that antigen. No T cells respond to the normal antigens displayed on dendritic cells, since the T cells that would have recognized those antigens have already been destroyed in the thymus.

How helper T cells are turned on (and off)

In the lymph nodes, helper T cells and antigen presenting cells interact in a complicated, sophisticated dance. When a helper cell and the antigen presenting cell bump into each other, a group of molecules lightly connects the two cells to each other. This connection lets the helper T cell scan the surface of the antigen presenting cell for the antigen it can recognize. If it doesn't see it, it simply lets go; the antigen is not present and there is no need for this helper T cell to take action. But if it does see its antigen, a number of molecular interactions take place, to ensure that the helper T cell responds in the right way.

The most important of these interactions is called "co-stimulation." During co-stimulation, a molecule (B7) on the antigen presenting cell connects to a molecule (CD28) on the helper T cell. Co-stimulation is very important because it determines how the helper T cell will respond. If a helper T cell sees its antigen, and gets the co-stimulatory signal, it acts as if the antigen were an invader, and begins to react against it. If, however, it sees its antigen without the costimulation, then it becomes completely unresponsive to that antigen now or at any point in the future. In essence, that particular helper T cell has been permanently turned off. This seems to be a way to turn off dangerous T cells which react to self but escaped education in the thymus. Some helper T cells may, however, be turned off in this way by cancer cells.

The first job of the newly stimulated helper T cell is to make many identical copies of itself (Figure22.1). The new helper T cells also begin to make proteins called cytokines.

Cytokines

Cytokines are the communication molecules of the immune system. They carry messages and instructions from one immune cell to another. There are many different cytokines. Many can stimulate the activity of immune system cells. A few inhibit the immune system. Cytokines also have activities outside the immune system. They are, for example, responsible for the fever and aches during infections such as the flu. The helper T cells are a particularly important source of cytokines. They make a cytokine called interleukin-2 which stimulates helper T cells to divide (the helper T cells actually stimulate their own cell division). They also make cytokines which help the other lymphocytes, the cytotoxic T cells and B cells, to respond to an antigen. Finally, they make some cytokines to stimulate the neutrophils, macrophages and Natural Killer cells to become more effective at their jobs. Several of these cytokines, as we will see in later chapters, are used in cancer treatment.

Turning on the rest of the immune system - the cytotoxic T cell responses

Cytokines from the newly-stimulated helper T cells help the cytotoxic T cells and B cells to turn themselves on. Like the helper T cells, cytotoxic T cells need input from several different sources. They need specific cytokines from the helper T cell. Each cytotoxic T cell must also find a body cell which is displaying the antigen it recognizes. This time, however, the antigen must be displayed in a molecule called the MHC class I molecule (Figure 22.2). Nearly all cells in the body carry MHC class I molecules on their surfaces; in these molecules, they show the cytotoxic T cells all of the proteins that can be found inside that cell. In a normal cell, these proteins would be self proteins, to which the cytotoxic T cells will not react. If, however, a cell is infected with a virus, it also displays pieces of virus on its surface. If it is a cancer cell, it may display altered proteins that should not be found in normal cells. One trick that some cancer cells use to avoid cytotoxic T cells is simply to stop making MHC I molecules (Baskar,1996; Kuby, 1997).

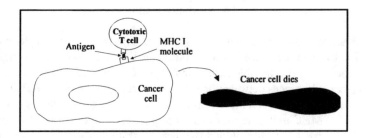

Figure 22.2. Cytotoxic T cells recognize cells which display "non-self" antigens in MHC I molecules, and kill them.

Like the helper cells, the cytotoxic T cells respond by dividing and making many copies of themselves. The new cells also turn into very efficient killer cells, which are now capable of turning around and killing any cells in the body which carry the antigen they recognize - including the one that helped to turn them on in the first place! They travel to any part of the body where cells are displaying their antigen, and destroy all of the abnormal cells.

It takes about a week for the T cell numbers to expand (Ahmed, 1996). During this time, the other cells of the immune system (the "innate immunity") are on their own, to control the invaders. Often, they don't do a very good job! After the expansion, there can be 100 to 5000 times as many cytotoxic T cells and up to 1200 more helper T cells as before (Ahmed, 1996). If an infection is taken care of, the excess T cells die over the next few weeks (Ahmed, 1996). A group of helper T cells and cytotoxic T cells, however, remains behind. These cells are called memory cells and are designed to respond very quickly and efficiently if the same invader tries to enter the body again. These memory cells are why a second exposure to a particular virus or bacterium often results in no symptoms at all.

The antibody response

When antibodies are needed, the B cells are stimulated. Like the cytotoxic T cells, the B cells need cytokines from the helper T cells. As you might expect, only B cells which see their antigens can respond. There are a few minor differences between the cytotoxic T cell and the B cell response. One difference is that the B cells do not need to see their antigens in any sort of MHC molecules; they can recognize an antigen which is simply floating past. Another minor difference is that stimulated B cells turn into two different types of cells: plasma cells, which make tremendous amounts of antibody and then die, and memory B cells, which make only a little antibody and are the reserves for the next infection. Antibodies have many roles in the immune response. They can prevent viruses from infecting cells. They mark invading bacteria and viruses and make them easier for macrophages and neutrophils to find. They can also tag abnormal cells for Natural Killer cells and macrophages to kill. Finally, they can work with other proteins of the immune system (called "complement") to burst bacterial cells.

The immune system responds differently
to different types of threats

The immune system does not respond identically to all invaders. An effective response to a virus, for example, will be very different than an effective response to a bacterium. There seem to be two basic patterns of responses. In one response, helper T cells and B cells are the major players and antibodies are the major products. This antibody response is particularly effective against invading organisms which live and reproduce outside the cells of the body, such as most bacteria. The other response is more effective against problems with normal cells of the body, such as a virus infection, or a cancer. In this response, called cell-mediated immunity, helper T cells, cytotoxic T cells, macrophages and Natural Killer cells are the major players. The products of this response are cytotoxic T cells and cytokines. Cytotoxic T cells destroy abnormal cells. Cytokines turn up the activity of Natural Killer cells and macrophages; these two cell types then become much more effective in killing abnormal cells.

These two types of responses are not mutually exclusive; usually, either an antibody response or cell-mediated immunity predominates, but is not the sole response. Which response dominates may, however, be very important. There is growing evidence that some infections are not cured because the body simply responds to an invading organism with the wrong type of immunity. In the next few chapters, we will look at how the immune system responds specifically to cancers - and how researchers are trying to make that response more effective.

Chapter 23

How the immune system kills cancer cells - and how the cancer fights back

The interaction between a cancer and the immune system is like a battleground. Although it might seem that it should be very one sided, with the immune system killing the helpless cancer cells, this turns out not to be the case. Instead, it is more like a pitched battle. The immune system destroys the cancer cells - and the cancer cells fight back.

How the immune system kills cancer cells

The immune system responds to most tumors by making antibodies and also by producing cell mediated immunity. The antibodies are of questionable value; cell mediated immunity, however, seems to be an important defense (Kuby, 1997).

Cell mediated immunity, you might recall, consists of cytotoxic T cells, Natural Killer cells, macrophages, and the cytokines which stimulate these cells. Natural Killer cells and cytotoxic T cells seem to be the most important defenses against cancers. Under ideal conditions, cytotoxic T cells are more efficient than Natural Killer cells. When cytotoxic T cells encounter their antigens, a single cell can turn into a hundred or more cells. The Natural Killer cell remains a single cell. There are, however, situations where Natural Killer cells can be very important. Other immune cells also seem to participate in defenses against cancer, although their importance is somewhat controversial. Macrophages often congregate around tumors, and their presence is sometimes associated with regression of the tumor (Kuby, 1997).

Antibodies, on the other hand, seem to have a Jekyll and Hyde approach to cancers. On the one hand, some antibodies can attach to antigens on the cancer cell's surface, and help macrophages, neutrophils and Natural Killer cells find the tumor and kill it. On the other hand, antibodies may hide the tumor from lymphocytes, by blocking the antigens that these cells must recognize (Kuby, 1997). An odd phenomenon can also take place, when antibodies attach to a tumor. In the presence of these antibodies, some tumors will sometimes discard their antigens and become invisible to the immune system (Kuby, 1997; Abbas, 1994).

How the tumor fights back

One of the best way to avoid the immune system is simply to hide, and cancer cells seem to do that quite well. Only a small percentage of their surface molecules may be different from normal, so it may be relatively easy for them to masquerade as normal cells. But they also have some more active ways of pretending not to be there. Cancer cells often carry reduced numbers of MHC I molecules (Baskar, 1996; Kuby, 1997). If the MHC I molecules are missing, the antigens are too, and the cytotoxic T cells can no longer recognize the tumor. Tumors can also cover themselves with normal molecules as a disguise. For example, some cancer cells can turn on the blood clotting system to hide themselves (Abbas, 1994). Blood clotting produces a tangled web of proteins known as fibrin; the tumors end up covered in a shell of fibrin (sometimes called a "fibrin cocoon") which blocks them from the immune cells. Finally, cancer cells seem to have ways of slipping away from the immune system - sometimes literally. Cancer cells are sometimes missing the "sticky" molecules (integrins) which help immune cells attach to their targets (Roitt, 1996).

But tumors don't just hide. In many cases, cancers seem to actively fight back against the immune system. Tumors suppress the immune system by producing a variety of chemicals, including some cytokines which suppress immunity (Roitt, 1996; Abbas, 1994). They also seem to produce abnormalities in antigen presenting cells and T cells . For example, some of the T cells at the tumor site have been turned off and are not responding to the tumor (Roitt, 1996).

Recently, researchers discovered that some melanomas can actually kill immune cells directly. They do this by displaying on their surfaces a molecule that triggers apoptosis (Hahne, 1996). This molecule, Fas L, attaches to Fas molecules on the surface of attacking T cells; this interaction prompts the T cell to commit suicide (Figure 23.1). With this surprising defense, the tumor cells have actually turned the tables on the T cells.

Ordinarily, T cells kill cancer cells by carrying FasL and instructing them to commit suicide. Most body cells have Fas but not FasL; they are, therefore, susceptible to being killed but cannot themselves kill. These cancer cells had, however, protected themselves from being killed by FasL. They had lost Fas while gaining FasL. This strategy enabled them to kill, but not to be killed. This discovery has opened up some new possibilities for fighting these cancers (Figure23.1). For example, blocking FasL on the tumors could protect the immune cells. On the other hand, putting Fas back on the tumor cells could make them susceptible to killing by immune cells again - or even make the cancer cells kill each other!

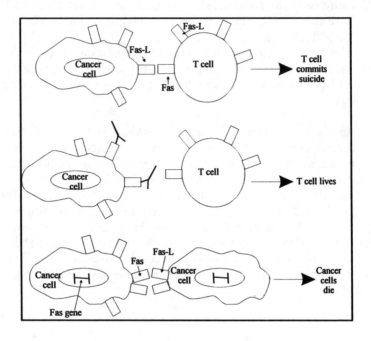

Figure 23.1. (a) Cancer cells carrying Fas-L can kill T cell. (B) If the Fas-L is blocked by antibodies, the T cell is protected. (C) If the gene for Fas could be put back into the cancer cells, their Fas - Fas-L interactions could kill each other.

The evolution of a tumor -
how the immune system helps to hide the tumor

There is one final problem in the battle between the immune system and the tumor, which may ultimately allow the tumor to win. The immune response against the cancer can be self-defeating; sometimes, it can make the tumor evolve into one that is less visible to the immune system (Abbas, 1994). In effect, it gives cells which hide from or attack the immune system a growth advantage. In any population of cancer cells, some cells are better able to avoid the immune system. Others are more easily killed. The immune response will kill the cells it can - but the others will escape and produce more cells. Gradually, the entire tumor population can become more resistant to the immune system. Some researchers think that this is part of the reason that, by the time most tumors are detected, the immune system doesn't seem to be doing a very good job of defense. In the next few chapters, we will look at some ways that researchers are trying to turn up the immune response, to give it the upper hand against tumors.

Chapter 24

Boosting the immune system to fight cancer

People with suppressed immune systems tend to get cancer more often. (Tuting, 1997) Organ transplant patients, who take drugs to stop immune reactions to the transplant, and AIDS patients have an increased risk for some types of cancer (Kuby, 1997). Some researchers, therefore, think that a healthy immune system may destroy some new cancers before they get a chance to grow. With most existing cancers, however, the immune system seems to be doing a rather poor job. Although immune cells are often seen around the tumor, this response is rarely effective. Nevertheless, there have been a few cases where melanoma skin cancers have spontaneously disappeared, and that disappearance seemed to be linked to an immune response (Bear, 1996; Gattoni-Celli, 1996; Tuting,1997). Some cancer researchers are, therefore, convinced that if they could effectively stimulate the immune system in cancer patients, the boosted immunity might help to destroy the cancer -- just as it apparently has in those few melanomas.

Lessons from early attempts

The first attempts to treat cancer by boosting the immune system occurred quite a long time ago, before very much was known about cancer. At first, researchers thought that cancer cells should look very foreign to the body. Naturally, they thought that cancers could be treated like other invaders such as bacteria or viruses. In 1895, researchers made the first attempt to treat tumors with antibodies, following a procedure sometimes used at the time for infections (Ben-Efraim, 1996). They made antibodies to a bone tumor and injected them into patients. They apparent saw some temporary decreases in tumor size, but the cancers promptly returned again. After many investigators had tried many experiments with antibodies, and been disappointed with the results, cancer researchers eventually became rather disillusioned with antibody treatment (Ben - Efraim, 1996). They concluded that either their preparations contained no antibodies which could attach only to tumor cells, or else that antibodies were not effective against cancer.

As researchers learned more about cancers, they began to realize that both answers were probably right. Antibodies don't seem to be very effective against cancer; T cells, Natural Killer cells, and macrophages seem to be much more important (Kuby, 1997). Cancer cells also look too much like "self" to the immune system. Although tumor cells may carry some unique or mutated proteins, most of their antigens are the same antigens found on normal cells. The early antibody mixtures would not have been able to distinguish between cancer cells and normal cells. Researchers also began to suspect that the body has a certain amount of tolerance even to unique tumor antigens. Tolerance means that immune cells ignore an antigen and do not react to it. It is normally a very good thing when it is directed at "self" antigens; otherwise, the immune system would destroy the rest of the body. But tolerance to cancer cells is not, of course, a positive attribute. A final problem was that the cancer cells themselves were able to suppress the immune system, and make any potential response even less effective (Musiani, 1997; Kuby, 1997; Abbas).

So now cancer researchers were faced with a tumor which doesn't look very dangerous to the immune system, and an immune system which has been turned down by the presence of the tumor. As a result, researchers have tried two different ways to enhance immune responses to cancer. One approach is to try to unmask the cancer cells to the immune system, using methods such as vaccination. The other is to try to boost the immune response, in general, using cytokines or other "non-specific immunostimulators".

Nonspecific immunostimulators

Some researchers think that the major problem with immune responses to tumors is a suppressed immune system rather than lymphocytes which cannot recognize cancer antigens. This idea is supported by the presence, in tumors, of lymphocytes and other immune cells which seem to be reacting to foreign antigens. If these researchers are right, then simply boosting the existing immune response should be an effective way to kill cancer cells. One way to increase existing immune reactions is to use "nonspecific immunostimulators."

Non-specific immunostimulators are substances which increase any and all immune responses that are occurring at the time; they do not select immune responses to a particular antigen. The first nonspecific immunostimulators to be used against cancer included whole bacteria and bacterial extracts. One commonly used bacterium is referred to as BCG, for Bacillus Calmette Guerin (Ben-Efraim, 1996). It is a weakened bacterium, used as a vaccine for tuberculosis in some parts of the world. Other bacteria, hormones made by the thymus (the organ where T cells mature) and some drugs (such as Levamisole) have also been used (Ben-Efraim, 1996). Nonspecific immunostimulators increase the activity of a variety of immune system cells such as lymphocytes and macrophages (Ben-Efraim, 1996).

Some temporary benefits have been seen with bacterial immunostimulators and Levamisole, but, as a whole, they have not been very effective (Ben-Efraim, 1996; Thurnher, 1997). One possible exception is the use of BCG, placed directly inside the urinary bladder, for the treatment of certain small bladder cancers (Berkow, 1992; DeBoer, 1997; Conti, 1994). In this case, BCG seems to act by increasing the production of cytokines and active immune cells in the urine. In other situations, BCG has only occasionally been effective (Ben - Efraim, 1996).

The function of nonspecific immunostimulators in cancer treatment?

Some authors suggest that nonspecific immunostimulators may find their niche not as a therapy which is used alone, but in combination with surgery, radiation, and chemotherapy (Ben-Efraim, 1996). One reason they may be ineffective alone is that a large tumor may simply be too much for the immune system to deal with. Immune responses might, however, be able to kill single cells or small groups of cells such as small metastasis. If other treatments can kill most of the cancer cells, nonspecific immunostimulators might be able to boost the immune system enough to mop up the rest of the cells. Surgery, radiation and chemotherapy also suppress the immune system, which may allow cancer cells to spread throughout the body during these treatments (Ben - Efraim, 1996). Nonspecific immunostimulators may be able to prevent that suppression. For example, giving Levamisole after treatment with the chemotherapy drug 5-fluorouracil can restore the activity of some immune cells (Johnkoski, 1996).

Treatment with cytokines

Many of the benefits of the bacterial immunostimulators may be due to their ability to stimulate cytokine production. Cytokines, you may recall, are the messenger molecules of the immune system. Many cytokines can make immune system cells become more active. Researchers have been very excited about using cytokines to treat cancer. They are not, however, easy to use. One problem is that they rarely have only one action in the body. For example, a single cytokine can slow the growth of cells, protect them against virus infections, stimulate Natural Killer cell activity, and have many other minor effects, depending on the cells being studied and the amount of cytokine that is used! It is difficult to pick out a specific reaction and find a single cytokine that does it, but does not have other side effects. To complicate matters further, cytokines often stimulate the production of other cytokines; the final effect may have as much to do with other cytokines as with the one actually given to a patient.

Cytokines, like many cancer treatments, can also be dangerous. When they are not given very carefully, they can kill. This might seem a little surprising, when cytokines are a natural product of the body. J.U. Gutterman (1994) points out, however, that cytokines are usually produced by the body to act locally. They are also very potent molecules, effective in very tiny quantities. Therefore, when they get into the blood in high amounts and travel throughout the body, they can sometimes be deadly. (In fact, some bacterial infections, such as toxic shock syndrome, actually kill people by stimulating excess cytokine production.) For example, tiredness, fever, weight and appetite loss are common when the cytokine interferon is given to cancer patients (Gutterman, 1994). Higher doses of some cytokines can cause life-threatening leaks in blood vessels, resulting in fluid in the lungs and other serious problems. For these reasons, many cytokines are given under very careful supervision, even sometimes in intensive care situations, where hospital personnel can quickly respond to life-threatening side effects. Cytokines have certainly found some niches in cancer treatment - but, like many other therapies, they must be used carefully.

Cytokines used for cancer treatment

The most common cytokines in cancer treatment seem to be interleukin-2 (IL-2) and the interferons. IL-2 mainly stimulates helper T cells to divide and produce other cytokines. The interferons, however, have many different effects in the body. They suppress cell growth, in general, but enhance many immune functions. They can, for example, stimulate Natural Killer cells and macrophages to become more effective, or increase the amount of MHC protein on tumor cells, making them more visible to the immune system. There are several types of interferons, called interferon α (alpha), interferon β (beta), and interferon γ (gamma); however, these cytokines share many of the same activities. Other cytokines have also been tried in cancer treatment, with varying success.

Cytokines in clinical trials

Cytokines have occasionally produced remissions in human cancers, although they rarely seem to result in spectacular cures (Musiani, 1997). Cytokines have probably been most effective for treating certain leukemias. Interferonα is particularly useful in chronic myelogenous leukemia (CML), a cancer of white blood cells (Gutterman, 1994). In this disease, a chromosome abnormality seems to prevent granulocytes from dying. The number of granulocytes in the blood increases, although at first these cells remain relatively normal. This stage of the disease lasts for a long time; however, in most people, it eventually progresses to leukemia. During the early phase, while the extra granulocytes are still fairly normal, interferon can suppress the cells carrying the abnormal chromosome. In the majority (75 percent) of patients, interferon treatment results in completely normal looking blood. In 20-25 percent of the patients, the disease may be completely cured; some regressions have lasted for at least 8 years. Unfortunately, once CML has progressed to actual leukemia, interferon treatment does not seem to be very effective.

Cytokines don't usually have such reliable results against most "solid tumors," cancers where masses of cells accumulate at one site (Gutterman, 1994). There have been successes, but most have been modest. For example, researchers report that 15-20 percent of melanomas respond to IL-2 treatment (Garbe, 1995; Philip, 1997) and 10-15 percent to interferon α (Garbe, 1995; Gutterman, 1994). When these two cytokines are used together, the results are slightly better (Garbe, 1995). Recently, a few small studies combined cytokines (interferon and IL-2) with conventional chemotherapy, with much improved results (Bear, 1996; Garbe, 1995). As many as half of the melanomas responded in some of these studies. These studies, however, contained relatively few patients; larger trials must still confirm the results. Some other skin cancers, including squamous cell carcinoma, basal cell carcinoma, Kaposi's sarcoma, and mycosis fungoides may also be sensitive to IL-2, or interferons (Gutterman, 1994; Garbe, 1995). In some cases, injecting the cytokine directly into the cancer may be the most effective treatment. Complete responses, with more than 80 percent of tumors regressing, have been reported when either Interferonα or interferon β were injected into some skin cancers (Garbe, 1995).

Cytokines are often used in kidney cancer, as well. These cancers tend to be resistant to treatment with chemotherapy, but are relatively responsive to cytokines. Unfortunately, these responses are not usually dramatic. For example, in one recent study, eleven patients were treated with Interferonα and IL-2 and a chemotherapy drug which stimulates the immune system (Wersall, 1995). One patient had a partial remission, the disease stopped progressing in four patients, and two patients had "minor responses". In general, 10 percent to 20 percent of kidney cancers seem to regress at least partially with cytokine treatment (Dillman, 1994b; Gutterman, 1994). Researchers are evaluating cytokines for the treatment of other cancers, as well. For example, interferons, IL-2, and a cytokine known as Tumor Necrosis Factor (TNF) are being tested in prostate cancers (Sokoloff, 1996).

Cytokines as molecular symphony conductors: shifting the immune response toward cell-mediated immunity

Cytokines do more than simply stimulate the immune system. They also influence whether the immune system will respond to an antigen mainly with cell mediated immunity or with antibodies. One new way to use cytokines is to promote cell-mediated immunity and redirect immune responses away from antibody production. One cytokine, interleukin-12 (IL-12), is particularly good at stimulating cell-mediated immunity. IL-12 has dramatically suppressed some tumors in mice (Brunda, 1995; Tahara, 1995). Phase I (safety) studies of IL-12 were recently started in humans (Brunda, 1995). Some new experiments have found that high doses of interferons may also be able to shift the response toward cell mediated immunity (Gallagher, 1997).

Getting cytokines into the right neighborhood - increasing effectiveness and decreasing side effects

As we have mentioned, a big problem with cytokine use is their toxicity. Sometimes, getting an effective dose of cytokines into the blood may be impossible; the side effects could kill the patient more surely than the cancer would. This problem may, in some cases, account for the less than stellar results seen with cytokines. Some researchers have tried to produce high concentrations of cytokines locally at the tumor site, instead of injecting a dose of cytokines into the blood. In mice, injecting some cytokines, including interferonγ and IL-2, into the area of the tumor may be able to stimulate a strong immune reaction against the tumor (Musiani, 1997). In some cases, cytokines have also been put into immune cells to deliver them to the tumor.

Are cytokines being tried too late?

One factor to keep in mind is that most clinical trials use cytokines late in the disease, after conventional treatment has failed. At this point, many mutations may be present in each cancer cell (Gutterman, 1994). Based on the results with chronic myelogenous leukemia and other diseases, some researchers suggest that this might be too late. Researchers speculate that cytokine treatments might be more effective if they were done early in cancers, when there are only a few mutations in the cells (Gutterman, 1994). Some have also suggested that cytokines such as interferon may also be effective in preventing precancerous areas from turning into cancers.

Chapter 25

Using immune cells and antibodies to treat tumors

Cytokines and other non-specific immunostimulators are injected into the body to stimulate immune cells. But sometimes conditions in the body may conspire to suppress this response. The tumor may be suppressing the immune system. Some of the interactions needed for lymphocyte stimulation may be missing. The immune cells and cytokines may not all be in the right place at the right time. To bypass these problems, some researchers have taken immune cells out of the body, stimulated them with cytokines in the laboratory, where conditions can be controlled, then returned them to the body.

Lymphokine activated killer cells

In the 1980s, one of the most exciting developments in cancer treatment was LAK (lymphokine activated killer) cell therapy (Kuby, 1997). (Lymphokine, incidentally, is just another name for some cytokines). LAK cells are lymphocytes from the patient's blood which have been taken out of the body and stimulated in the laboratory by cytokines. LAK cells seem to be a mixture of cells; Natural Killer cells may be the most important. LAK cells are very efficient cancer cell killers. During LAK cell therapy, lymphocytes are collected from the patient's blood, treated in the laboratory with cytokines (usually IL-2 and interferonγ), then returned to the body with an additional dose of IL-2. The doses of IL-2 used in LAK cell therapy are fairly high, so side effects are common with this treatment (Hayes, 1995). In some experiments, giving LAK cells and IL-2 directly in the vicinity of the tumor, rather than into the blood, could reduce the side effects of treatment (Hayes, 1995).

The first experiments using LAK cell therapy looked very promising, particularly in melanomas and kidney cancers (Sussman, 1994). As results have accumulated from clinical trials, however, researchers have been disappointed. LAK cells are very effective at killing tumor cells grown in the laboratory and in animal models, but they have been less effective than hoped in human patients (Azuma, 1994). In fact, some recent experiments seem to show that the benefits of LAK therapy are probably due to the cytokines alone. In these studies, there was no difference in the response rates (15-20 percent) between cancer patients given LAK cells and IL-2, and patients given only IL-2 (Bear, 1996; Dillman 1994b; Philip, 1997).

One problem may be that LAK cells don't find their way effectively to the site of the tumor (Azuma, 1994). Some new technologies may, however, be able to guide the LAK cells to the tumor. In other cases, injecting LAK cells and IL-2 directly into the tumor may be more promising. In several recent experiments, researchers tried local LAK cell therapy in brain cancer. In one study, 10 patients (who had brain cancers which returned after conventional treatment) received LAK cells and IL-2 in the fluid that bathes the brain, the cerebrospinal fluid, or directly into the tumor (Sankhla, 1996). Only two patients, however, had partial responses to the treatment, and the responses were not long lasting. In another attempt, LAK cells and IL-2 were injected directly into brain tumors, with equally poor results (Boiardi, 1994). Some patients responded at first; however, eighteen months later, survival was no better than would have been expected in patients treated conventionally (Boiardi, 1994). In a third study, however, repeated injections of LAK cells and IL-2 into the tumor (rather than a one-time dose), had somewhat better results (Hayes, 1995). In this study, patients survived for significantly longer than expected. Average survival for patients treated with chemotherapy was 25 weeks, but average survival was 53 weeks with LAK and IL-2. One problem that does muddy the results of this trial is that six of the patients had additional surgery or chemotherapy after the immune treatments, which may have contributed to the good results.

Tumor infiltrating lymphocytes

A newer approach is to extract lymphocytes which are found inside or around the tumor and stimulate them in the laboratory (Sussman, 1994). Since these "tumor infiltrating lymphocytes" (TILs) are presumably already reacting to the cancer, they should be more effective than cells from the blood. TILs are stimulated in the laboratory like LAK cells; however, in this case, they are stimulated with tumor antigens or with other treatments that work on T cells. They are then are returned to the patient. One promising result is that, unlike LAK cells, TILs do seem to return to the tumors (Hermann, 1995). TILs have induced some tumor rejections in animal models and are currently being tested in humans (Kuby, 1997; Sussman, 1994). In some early trials in melanomas, TILs appear to be more effective than LAK cells (Bear, 1996).

TILs have also been used to deliver cytokines to the tumor, since they return to the tumor after being re-injected into the body. They are extracted as usual, but genes for cytokines are put into the cells before they are returned. The TILs should then produce extra cytokines, which may be able to stimulate not only the TILs, but also any other immune cells reacting to the tumor. Because the production of the cytokines is localized to the tumor, there are fewer side effects (Hermann, 1995). In fact, high doses of cytokines can be seen at the tumor in this form of therapy. These doses have been much higher than would be possible (without killing the patient) if cytokines were simply injected into the bloodstream (Hermann, 1995). Genetically modified TILs carrying IL-2 or tumor necrosis factor have had some benefit for patients with melanomas and kidney cancers (Hermann, 1995).

Increasing T cell responses inside the body -
Increasing T cell activity by increasing antigen presentation

Some researchers think that T cells might not react to cancer antigens because they are not getting the antigen presentation that they need (Anon, 1998a). One way to get around this problem is to stimulate T cells outside the body and return them, as in TIL treatment. This treatment, however, ignores the many lymphocytes that are still inside the body and which may be useful against tumors. In some new experiments, however, researchers are trying to stimulate the antigen presenting cells, instead of the T cells, outside the body (Anon, 1998a). They have extracted antigen presenting cells, given them tumor antigens to present, then re-injected them into animals. In one very small study at Stanford University, four human cancer patients were also given this treatment (Anon, 1998a). One patient had a complete response to this treatment, two responded partially, and the fourth responded briefly before his tumor again began to grow. Researchers have been encouraged by these results, and are continuing to test this treatment in cancer patients.

Unfortunately, such manipulations are cumbersome and expensive, because they must be done individually for each patient. TILs, LAK cell therapy, and stimulation of antigen presenting cells, share this disadvantage. Recent advances in our knowledge of T cell stimulation have, however, spawned a promising new technique which may be much simpler.

Manipulation of T cell co-stimulation

You might remember that, when helper T cells respond to an antigen, at least two things must happen. They must see their antigen and they must receive a second signal, called co-stimulation. Co-stimulation occurs when a molecule on the helper T cell called CD28 attaches to a molecule on the antigen presenting cell called B7 (Pardoll, 1996; Williams, 1996). Together, the antigen interaction and the CD28/B7 interaction turn on the T cell (Figure 25.1).

Recently, biologists have discovered that B7 can also attach to a different partner, called CTLA-4 (Figure 25.1), to turn off the T cell (Williams, 1996). This interaction seems to be one way the body keeps immune responses under control. When T cells first respond, they do not have CTLA-4, so the T cells are turned on. After T cells have been reacting for a time, they make CTLA-4; the newly made CTLA-4 can attach more firmly than CD28 to B7 and replaces CD28 as B7's partner. This turns the immune response off. This seems to be a good way to turn off short-term responses, such as immune reactions in an infection, where the invader is quickly eliminated. In cancer, however, some T cells may be turned off although the cancer is still present.

Cancer researchers have speculated that blocking CTLA-4 might leave more B7 free to interact with CD28, and so enhance immune responses (Figure 25.1). In some very early experiments, it seems that this treatment might work. D.R. Leach and colleagues injected mice with antibodies which attached to CTLA-4 and prevented it from attaching to B7 (Pardoll, 1996; Williams, 1996). This treatment did, in fact, increase the immune response to the tumors.. The danger of this treatment, however, is that it may prevent immune responses to other antigens from being turned off as well. This could eventually result in immune reactions against body tissues by the overstimulated T cells. Fortunately, there has not yet been any sign of this in these experiments (Pardoll, 1996).

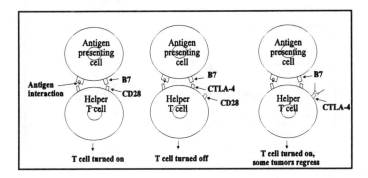

Figure 25.1. Helper T cells are turned on when B7 attaches to CD28, then turned off when B7 attaches to CTLA-4. Blocking CTLA-4 with antibodies can turn the T cell back on.

Antibodies revisited- treatment with monoclonal antibodies

The first attempts to treat cancer were with antibodies. These experiments, as we saw earlier, were not very effective. One of the problems was that natural antibody preparations contain antibodies which react against a tremendous variety of antigens. These early antibody preparations reacted to both normal cells and cancer cells. The answer to this problem came with the development of a technique to produce monoclonal antibodies, antibodies which are all identical. Monoclonal antibodies can be made to a single antigen found only on tumor cells; these antibodies can then specifically find and attach to cancer cells, while ignoring normal cells (Figure 25.2). Newer "humanized" monoclonal antibodies (chapter 11) may be even more promising.

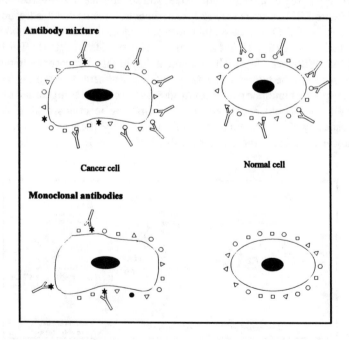

Figure 25.2. Monoclonal antibodies can attach to a single antigen found on cancer cells, but antibody mixtures usually attach to both normal cells and cancer cells.

When monoclonal antibodies were first developed, the end of cancer seemed to be in sight. When that hope didn't come true, there was disappointment and disillusionment, and many researchers abandoned antibody techniques. But monoclonal antibodies may not be dead yet, as an effective cancer treatment. We have already discussed new techniques which use antibodies as tools to block growth factors, or to bring poisons directly to tumor cells. The antibodies used for these techniques are monoclonal antibodies. Other new techniques, such as bispecific antibodies (discussed below), are approaching cancer treatment in new ways. Finally, the simple view that cell-mediated immunity is important, but antibodies are not, may not turn out to be the whole story.

In some situations, researchers think that cell mediated immunity and antibodies may both fight cancer (Baskar, 1996). For example, stimulation of the immune system in ways that are expected to produce antibodies rather than cell mediated immunity can sometimes enhance tumor rejection (Baskar, 1996). In this case, even plain monoclonal antibodies, without attached poisons or unique activities, might sometimes have a role to play. Such plain monoclonal antibodies have enjoyed some successes in animal models of cancer (Hall, 1995). Unfortunately, they haven't looked as good in human cancer patients (Hall, 1995). A 1994 review of monoclonal antibody treatment found that, although side effects were few, there seemed to be no proven benefit in either cancers of the blood or solid tumors (Dillman, 1994a).

More recent trials have had some mild successes, but also some failures. For example, in some relatively large clinical trials, patients with cancers of the pancreas did not seem to benefit from monoclonal antibody treatment; they neither survived longer nor had more remissions (Friess, 1997). Other studies, however, have been more encouraging. One recent study may be the first really convincing study of monoclonal antibodies in human patients. In this clinical trial, monoclonal antibodies were used in patients with colon cancer, after the primary tumor was treated with conventional therapies (Schneider-Gadicke, 1995). Antibody treatment decreased the death rate by 30 percent, and decreased cancer recurrence by 27 percent. The benefits were similar to those that would be expected if radiotherapy or chemotherapy were used to treat metastasis, but monoclonal antibody treatment had fewer side effects. This study gives weight to an idea that monoclonal antibodies may be most effective used as a part of early treatments, rather than as a last ditch effort after chemotherapy has failed (Schneider-Gadicke, 1995). It may also point out that all monoclonal antibodies are not the same.

Bispecific antibodies -
two attachment sites are better than one

Bispecific antibodies are antibody molecules which can attach to two antigens. Normal antibodies have two attachment sites for antigens, but ordinarily these two sites are identical. Bispecific antibodies have been engineered in the laboratory so that the two sites are different: one will attach to one antigen and the other will attach to a different antigen. These antibodies can attach either to two different cells or to two different antigens on one cell. Sometimes, these antibodies are made to attach to a greater variety of cancer cells, or to attach more tightly to some cancer cells. Another, more interesting, use is to bring immune system cells (usually Natural Killer cells and cytotoxic T cells) to the cancer. For example, they have been helpful in guiding LAK cells to tumors (Saijyo, 1996; Azuma, 1994) and may increase the effectiveness of LAK therapy.

Other bispecific antibodies have been able to gather human immune cells to the site of the tumor after antibody treatment alone (Renner, 1995). In some cases, mice with even advanced tumors have had complete regressions of their tumors after treatment with bispecific antibodies. Bispecific antibodies which can attach to the HER-2/neu protein (a growth factor on cancer cells) and also to macrophages, Natural Killer cells or neutrophils have been effective in increasing the survival of mice with ovarian cancer (Disis, 1997). They have recently been tested in humans safety (phase I) trials and appeared to be relatively safe (Disis, 1997). Some "minor" clinical responses were also seen in these tumors.

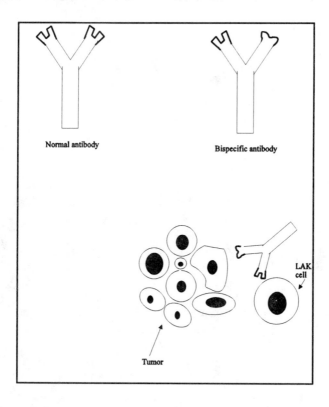

Figure 25.3. Bispecific antibodies can attach to two different antigens and can guide immune cells to a tumor.

Chapter 26

Cancer Vaccines

At the end of the 20th century, it is difficult to imagine life without vaccines. Because of vaccines, such terrible diseases as polio, smallpox, rabies and tetanus no longer haunt our lives. Most of us escape such childhood illnesses as measles, mumps, and rubella. Whooping cough and diphtheria are just names, when they once were common and dreaded diseases. Someday, some researchers hope, vaccines may help cure cancer, as well.

How most vaccines work

Vaccines against microorganisms such as bacteria or viruses work by mimicking a natural immune response. Before it has been exposed to a microorganism, the immune system has only a few lymphocytes which are capable of responding to that organism. These lymphocytes are in a resting state. When the body is infected by the organism for the first time, it takes a week or two to turn on the lymphocytes and generate enough new cells to take care of an invading organism. Meanwhile, of course, the organism is destroying cells and generally wreaking havoc in the body; in other words, causing an illness. Ultimately, the number of active lymphocytes rises, the invader is brought under control and killed by the immune system, and the disease ends. Most of the expanded pool of lymphocytes dies, but some remain behind as memory cells. These memory lymphocytes are long-lived cells which patrol for the organism, and generate a much faster and more effective immune response the next time it tries to invade.

Vaccination exposes the immune system to a weakened form of the disease organism, to generate memory lymphocytes against it. The vaccine organisms cannot cause disease, but can provoke an immune response. For example, a killed virus might be used, instead of the live organism. (Figure, 26.1) Sometimes, vaccines are made with only a few antigens from the organism; proteins can be used to stimulate a good immune response. Later when the real disease organism tries to invade, there will already be memory cells, which will eliminate the organism before it can ever get a good foothold in the body. The person will never even know that the invader was there.

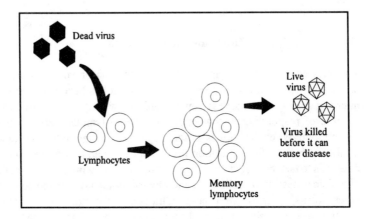

Figure 26.1. Vaccination exposes the system to a weakened antigen and generates memory lymphocytes, which can defend the body against later invasions by the same organism

How cancer vaccines work

At the moment, most cancer vaccines are designed to be used in people who already have cancer. This is an unusual use of vaccines, since ordinarily someone who has the disease is being exposed to plenty of antigen, and vaccination at that point will do no good. In cancer, however, the vaccines have a slightly different purpose. Possibly because cancer cells are so similar in some ways to normal body cells (Ben-Efraim, 1996), the immune response against them seems to be weak or limited (Melief, 1996; Mastrangelo, 1996; Baskar, 1996). Cancer vaccines are designed to alert the immune system to the invader, to boost the immune response to the point where it will be effective. In effect, they are a wake up call to the cells of the immune system.

Cancer antigens

To make an effective vaccine, researchers must find antigens that immune cells will react to. For some cancers, this may not be too difficult. For example, cancers initiated by a virus, such as cervical cancers, can carry virus proteins on their surfaces (Melief, 1996). Other cancers, however, may look too much like normal cells to the immune system. Although some cancer cells carry mutated proteins on their surfaces, others simply make too much of certain normal antigens (Baskar, 1996; Melief, 1996). Other cancer antigens come from genes which were active before birth, but have been turned off in normal cells in the adult.

During an immune response, B and T cells do not react equally to all antigens. For example, if a vaccine contained a mixture of proteins, the immune system would react strongly to some of them, more weakly to others. Researchers often try to identify the antigens the immune system will respond to, then use those antigens to make vaccines. One approach is to find patients with documented tumor regressions which were probably caused by the immune system - then discover which antigens are recognized by T cells from those patients (Mastrangelo, 1996). Researchers have recently used T cells from patients with melanomas to identify a group of proteins called the MAGE antigens. MAGE proteins are not found on normal adult cells (with the exception of a few cells such as those which make sperm). They are, however, found on some tumor cells including a number of melanomas, lung cancers, bladder cancers, and head and neck tumors (Mastrangelo, 1996; Williams, 1996). Currently, researchers are trying to use T cells to identify antigens from ovarian and breast cancers (Linehan, 1996). Researchers hope that these newly-discovered antigens might make good vaccines.

Cancer vaccines in the clinic and in preclinical trials

How do you catch the attention of a lymphocyte that's ignoring an antigen and stimulate it to respond? One way to do it is to give the antigen in an unusual form. Another is to give the antigen with a stimulant which can boost the immune response. One important immune stimulant is called an adjuvant. It is a mixture of chemicals or pieces of bacterial organisms which boosts an immune response to antigens. Adjuvants seem to work by keeping the antigens at the site of the injection longer, or by stimulating the antigen presenting cells. They are included with most vaccines. Cytokines have also been used as immune stimulants for vaccines.

Vaccines made by modifying and re-injecting tumor cells from the patient

Many cancer vaccines are simply killed whole cancer cells. Usually, these cancer cells are taken from each individual patient, killed or otherwise prevented from dividing and re-injected as a vaccine (Mastrangelo, 1996; Baskar, 1996). Experiments using unmodified tumor cells in patients with existing melanomas have generally been disappointing (Mastrangelo, 1996). For example, only five complete responses and six partial responses were seen among 56 patients in two studies (Mastrangelo, 1996). It seems that simply injecting whole tumor cells, with an adjuvant, is not very effective in stimulating the immune system.

In newer vaccines, the cancer cells have often been modified to increase their visibility to the immune system. Sometimes, researchers can make the immune system respond to an antigen that it ignores by giving the antigen in an unusual form. A common way to do this is to hook on a tiny chemical called a hapten. The hapten seems to unmask the rest of the antigen to the immune system. If all goes well, when the immune system responds to the hapten modified cells, some lymphocytes will also respond to the unmodified cancer cells remaining in the body (Figure 26.2)

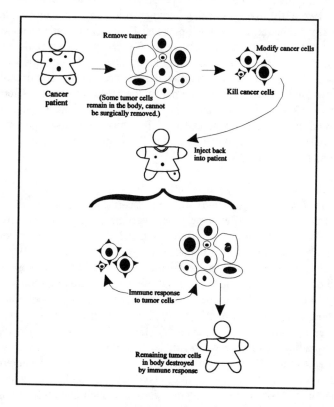

Figure 26.2. Whole cell vaccines can be made by modifying cancer cells from a patient then re-injecting them to generate an immune response.

Although hapten-modified vaccines seem to work better than most unmodified tumor cell, the majority have had only modest benefits. One recent hapten-modified vaccine, however, was remarkably effective (Berd, 1997). This vaccine was tested in a clinical trial for melanoma patients with metastasis in lymph nodes. In this trial, patients first had surgery to remove their tumors. Cancer cells from each patient were modified by haptens and killed, then the modified cells were re-injected into the patient. Thirty six of 62 patients (58 percent) with metastasis in one lymph node were still alive, two and a half to six years after treatment. Five of 15 patients (33 percent) with metastasis in two lymph nodes were still alive. A startling finding in this study is that older patients actually did better than younger patients: 47 percent of patients under 50 years old were expected to survive for 5 years, but 71 percent over 50 were expected to survive for that time. In other trials with this vaccine (Sato, 1996), the researchers found that the vaccine could prolong survival in later stages of melanoma, but their results were not as good as in patients with earlier cases. They also found that many melanomas seemed to make a cytokine called IL-10 which suppresses the immune response, and suggested that inhibiting IL-10 might improve the vaccine results in late stage disease.

Another way to modify tumor antigens is by infecting cancer cells with viruses (Mastrangelo, 1996). In some cases, animals have developed immunity to tumors after being given a vaccine made from virus infected cancer cells (Schmidt, 1996). In humans, however, virus-modified vaccines have not been particularly successful (Mastrangelo, 1996;). A new technique may promise some improvement in these results. One way to modify tumor cells is to put small pieces of a virus into the tumor's MHC I molecules before they are injected back into the patient. The new technique, called transloading, is simply a more efficient way to get virus pieces into the MHC I molecules (Schmidt, 1996). In the first test of transloading, a vaccine was made by loading small proteins from the influenza virus directly into MHC I molecules of either melanoma or colon cancer cells. These vaccines cured seven of eight mice with very small metastasis. The researchers suggest that such good results may be routinely possible, if enough virus peptides can be delivered into tumor cells.

Cytokine enhanced vaccines

There have been at least 30 trials where cytokine genes were put into cancer cells and given to mice as vaccines (Mastrangelo, 1996). Most of these tests were "challenge" experiments: the vaccine was given first, then the animals were given tumor cells and monitored to see whether the tumor cells would grow or be eliminated (Mastrangelo, 1996; Davis, 1996). Eliminating established tumors, unfortunately, is a bit more difficult, although there have been some successes in animal studies (Mastrangelo, 1996; Baskar, 1996; Ben-Efraim, 1996; Davis, 1996). One recent study suggests that some of the vaccines may not have worked simply because not enough of the cytokine genes made it into the cancer cells (Schmidt, 1997). These researchers were able to put cytokine genes (IL-2 or GM-CSF) more efficiently into cancer cells; their vaccines cured 80% of mice with existing small metastasis.

Cytokine-modified cancer vaccines are currently being tested in human clinical trials (Tuting, 1997). Some results from these studies are available. So far, they do not appear to be particularly impressive. In one case, although melanoma vaccines with IL-2 had good responses in animals, human clinical trials with melanoma cells with IL-2 genes were not very successful (Parmiani, 1996). The response of patients to the vaccine was described as "weak", and few patients generated cytotoxic T cells in response to the vaccine. In another phase I trial, 20 melanoma patients received their own tumor cells back, with an interferon gene inserted (Abdel-Wahab, 1997). Although the vaccine seemed to be safe enough, only eight of the 13 patients who completed the treatment had a measurable immune response to the vaccine. Two of these patients experienced a clinical regression, while the tumor shrank temporarily in two other patients, then returned. The authors of the study suggest trying the vaccine in patients with less advanced cancers.

Protein and peptide vaccines

One problem with using whole cell vaccines is the labor and expense involved in collecting cancer cells from each individual patient, growing them in the laboratory, and modifying them before use as a vaccine (Mastrangelo, 1996). Another problem is that all patients may not have enough tumor cells to use in a vaccine, or a particular individual's tumor cells may refuse to grow in the laboratory. To get around these problems, some researchers have made vaccines from proteins collected from tumor cells.

The crudest of these vaccines are made by collecting cancer cells from different patients, breaking the cells up, and collecting the pieces (Mastrangelo, 1996). One problem with such vaccines is that most of the proteins in the mixture are normal proteins and are not unique to the cancer (Mastrangelo, 1996). Another problem is that some normal proteins (such as MHC molecules) are different between individuals. The recipient of the vaccine may have his or her immune system so busy responding to the normal proteins it considers to be foreign, that it completely ignores the cancer antigens (Mastrangelo, 1996).

Researchers are, therefore, using new information about cancer antigens to select specific proteins to generate an immune response. Many of the new vaccines use even smaller pieces of proteins, called peptides. Researchers are trying to identify the peptides that cytotoxic T cells and helper T cells tend to respond to, and include only those peptides in a vaccine. In this way, they hope to stimulate effective cell mediated immunity to cancer cells.

In animal studies of cancer, peptide vaccines have enjoyed at least limited success (Melief, 1996). In humans, however, peptide vaccines have not resulted in many dramatic remissions. Several different studies have tested various peptides from melanomas in human cancer patients. In one study, cytotoxic T cells were made in response to the vaccine, but none of the patients' cancers responded (Melief, 1996). A different peptide resulted in three very minor responses among 23 patients (Mastrangelo, 1996) In a third study, six patients with advanced melanomas received weekly injections of six different peptides (Jaeger, 1996). Once again, cytotoxic T cells were made in five of the patients. This time, however, the cancers also stopped growing in two patients. No major regressions were, however, seen. A new vaccine against the melanoma antigen MAGE-3 may, however, be more promising (Mastrangelo, 1996). This vaccine was recently tested in the clinic in a phase I (safety) trial. No responses were really expected, since the concern was mainly safety and the vaccine was being tested without an adjuvant. One out of 12 patients given this vaccine had a complete response and two had partial responses (Mastrangelo, 1996). Other protein and peptide vaccines are also being evaluated (Mastrangelo, 1996).

Naked DNA vaccines

Some very unusual vaccines are nothing more than pieces of DNA. In the early 1990s, a startling experiment showed that a simple piece of circular DNA, unprotected in any way, could be incorporated into body cells and start making proteins - just by injecting the DNA into muscle or skin (Taubes, 1997; Conry, 1996). Surprisingly enough, this process was fairly efficient; the DNA actually got into cells better than when researchers deliberately try to put genes into cells in the laboratory! Since then, naked DNA vaccines have been used to generate immunity to a large number of microorganisms and also to tumor cells in mouse models (Conry, 1996).

Researchers speculate that some DNA vaccines might be able to stimulate immunity to tumor antigens by showing them to immune cells in a new environment, namely in muscle or skin cells. Other types of DNA vaccines, injected directly into tumor cells, may make these cells more visible to the immune system.

Naked DNA vaccines are very new and there are not yet many laboratories using them as cancer vaccines. They have, however, been effective in several cases. DNA vaccines have been used in mice who have too many copies of the HER-2/neu growth factor gene (Disis, 1997). These mice typically develop breast tumors when they are 6-7 months old. Vaccination could, however, slow the development and growth of these tumors. Naked DNA vaccines may soon be tested in humans as well. Researchers are planning to use naked DNA to boost immunity to "carcinoembryonic antigen," a cancer antigen, in colon cancer patients (Conry, 1996).

Side effects of vaccines

Perhaps the greatest fear with cancer vaccines is that some of them may stimulate the development of immune responses against normal cells. Vaccines which use antigens unique to tumor cells do not run this risk. Other vaccines, however, are made using normal proteins found in excess on cancer cells. The *HER-2*/neu gene, for example, is overactive in some cancer cells and its protein is being tested as a cancer vaccine. The HER-2 protein can, however, be found in small amounts on normal cells as well. One of the fears with the HER-2/neu vaccines is that people might develop immune responses which would damage normal cells as well as cancer cells (Disis, 1997). Such immune responses, once started, would be extremely difficult to stop; diseases where the immune system reacts to normal cells, called autoimmune diseases, can cause severe damage to the body. Fortunately, no evidence of such problems has been seen in people with naturally occurring immune responses to HER-2/neu (Disis, 1997). Researchers hope, therefore, that such vaccines will be safe.

Other vaccines may contain antigens which were present during fetal development and have been reactivated in cancer cells. Such vaccines carry a risk of damage to a developing child, if a cancer patient is cured and later becomes pregnant (Disis, 1997). Such fears may be real. In one small study, ten mice were vaccinated with HER-2/neu, then allowed to become pregnant. Seven of the ten pregnant mice miscarried or had fewer pups than expected (Disis, 1997). Many chemotherapy treatments used for cancer treatment cause sterility; therefore, such fears may be more theoretical than real for most human cancer patients (Disis, 1997). Such immune responses might, however, limit some vaccines from ever being used as a preventative for cancer.

Chapter 27

Gene therapy - a glimpse into the future

Perhaps the most intriguing idea to come out of cancer research has been the possibility that we might someday be able to treat cancer as a genetics problem, and simply replace defective genes like parts in a car. We could replace defective tumor suppressor genes and stop or slow the tumor's growth. We could also target oncogenes and turn them off, perhaps even making the cancer cells revert to normal. Maybe someday an important part of cancer treatment will be to catalogue the genetic defects that exist in a person's cancer, and make a cocktail of genes to correct the most important of those defects. Although this is still a fantasy, in some ways we have progressed remarkably toward this goal. In many others, we are still a long way off. In this section, we will look at where we are and at the obstacles that stand in the way of the genetic cure of cancer.

The first step toward this goal is, of course, the identification of the defective genes in cancer cells. As we discussed in chapter 4 and 5, we now know many of the players in cancer, and are rapidly finding others. We know about tumor suppressor genes such as *p53* and the retinoblastoma gene. "Oncogenes" are no longer merely mysterious cancer genes: we now recognize them individually as defective growth factor receptors, defective cell signaling proteins, altered cell cycle controllers, and many others. We see patterns of mutations in certain cancers. We also realize that cancers are individual: each person's cancer has a specific set of mutations and accumulates more, as it grows. While we are far from the identification of every oncogene or tumor suppressor, or even from a complete knowledge of how cells work, those goals no longer seem impossible. Gene therapy in human patients is in fact, beginning.

How do you do gene therapy?

The basic approach to gene therapy is quite simple: find a gene, make copies of it, and deliver those copies into the cells. The technical aspects and practicalities are, however, quite complex. It is no simple matter even to find a gene! There are large textbooks devoted to genetic engineering; we will only take a brief peek at the process.

The first part of this process, finding and making copies of a gene, is a technique used every day in laboratories at every major university and biotechnology company. Perhaps the most difficult part of the process is finding a gene involved in a particular type of cancer and making the first copy. Biologists who do such work must be good detectives; too often, the clues they have to follow may point at several genes or at entire segments of a chromosome containing many genes. Once the gene has been found, making copies is routine (although the technical details can sometimes be quite frustrating).

Once the gene has been found, the first decision is whether to take the cells out of the body and insert the gene in the laboratory, then return them to the patient - or to deliver the gene into the patient's body and ensure that it gets to the right cells. The first approach, inserting the genes into cells in the laboratory, is technically the simpler of the two approaches. In cancer treatment, it has mainly been used to make genetically engineered tumor vaccines. In this technique, cells are usually taken from the patient during surgery and kept alive in the laboratory. Genes are inserted into the cells. The cells which have incorporated the gene are identified and separated from the cells which have not. (When cancer cells are used, the cells are then treated so that they cannot continue to divide and grow.) Finally, they are returned to the patient.

The second approach takes the gene to the cancer cells. With this technique, researchers hope to put genes into cancer cells still in the body and destroy them. The gene is simply isolated, put into some sort of delivery system, and inserted into the body to seek out the cancer cells. It sounds simpler, but is actually more technically complex. The greatest difficulty in this approach is with the delivery system. The gene must find, infect and remain permanently active in the cancer cells throughout the body. This, we shall see, is not an easy thing to do.

The critical step in both approaches is getting the gene into the cells and, ultimately, into the chromosome. At the moment, there are a number of more or less efficient ways to get genes into cells. Two of these techniques can be used either in the laboratory, or injected directly into the body of a cancer patient. In one technique, genes are mixed into small clumps of fats called liposomes, which help to transport the genes across cell membranes and into the cell (Hermann, 1995; Davis, 1996; Crystal, 1995). In the other, specially modified viruses can carry genes into the cells they infect (Hermann, 1995; Davis, 1996; Crystal, 1995). These gene delivery viruses have been made harmless by removing some of their essential genes, so that they cannot hijack the cell to make more virus particles. All they are capable of doing is infecting a single cell and delivering the target gene to it. Both liposomes and virus delivery systems are being used in cancer gene therapy.

A sobering pause - practical problems with gene therapy

In spite of media enthusiasm, gene therapy for cancer will probably not become common anytime soon (although "suicide genes," discussed below, may be an exception). Although there have been gene therapy experiments in humans for the last five years, there have been few published reports of successful clinical trials. There are yet a number of problems to be overcome. Perhaps it would be well to keep them in mind as we discuss gene therapy.

Possibly the greatest difficulty is to get enough genes into cells, and make sure that the genes continue to function. At the moment, it is impossible to ensure that each cell will get a copy of the gene. Even when genes are mixed with cells in the laboratory under ideal conditions, only one in every 100 to 10,000,000 cells will permanently insert the gene into its chromosome (Hermann, 1995). When genes are placed inside the human body, conditions are much less controlled and the possibilities of success even less. If the gene is a tumor suppressor gene, intended to replace a defective copy of the tumor suppressor in cancer cells, this will obviously never work. One in every hundred or so cancer cells might stop dividing, but that still leaves 99 or more to continue unchecked. To make things even worse, sometimes new genes in cells will simply be shut off after a time, never to function again (Hermann, 1995). This has happened with gene therapy in patients: new genes have sometimes functioned for a few weeks, then mysteriously stopped working (Hermann, 1995).

A second problem is making certain that the genes get into the right cells (Hermann, 1995). When cells are taken out of the body and modified, this is not a great problem; a researcher can control exactly which cells are exposed to the gene. If the gene is, however, put into the body and expected to get to the right cells, targeting becomes a lot trickier. How do you find the cancer cells in a sea of other cells? And, if the gene is one that causes cells to self-destruct, how do you keep that gene out of normal cells? It doesn't look like this problem is insoluble - but the solutions are still in the early stages. For example, liposomes can be tagged with molecules that deliver the gene specifically to some cells and not to others (although this process is not yet perfect) (Hermann, 1995). Most gene therapy, so far, has gotten around this problem by simply injecting the gene (in its virus or liposomes) directly into the tumor.

A third issue is safety. When genes get put into chromosomes, they do not always go where we want them to go (Crystal, 1995; Hermann, 1995). A worst case scenario is the gene that jumps inside a normal cell gene, destroying it, or turns on an oncogene and makes the cancer cells more malignant rather than less so. Worse yet, if it accidentally lands in a normal cell, it could potentially initiate a second cancer. A unique problem with virus delivery systems is the possibility that the virus might eventually get together with another defective virus from another source and exchange pieces (Crystal, 1995; Hermann, 1995). If the viruses are missing different parts, the combination might make a new, infectious virus, which could cause disease. So far, there have been no signs of either problem in experiments (Crystal, 1995). Nevertheless, biologists are continuing to work on gene delivery systems to minimize the chances of giving the patient either new cancers or new viruses along with the gene therapy.

There have, however, been other safety problems. For example, in one clinical trial, unexpected immune reactions led to problems (Crystal, 1995). In this trial, genes were placed in brain tumors, carried inside cells which acted simply as inert carriers. The immune system reacted to the foreign cells and created symptoms of brain toxicity in these patients. Absolutely no problems had been seen in preclinical studies with the same therapy in laboratory animals (Crystal, 1995). The immune system can also react against virus delivery systems. This immune response could eliminate the virus - and the gene therapy carried with it (Crystal, 1995). It could also cause disease, or at least discomfort, by damaging normal cells.

Current trials of gene therapy

Considering all of the problems mentioned above, it should not come as a surprise that much of the current research is trying to make gene therapy more efficient and safe. At the same time, some trials of gene therapy are also beginning. Most of these studies have been preclinical trials, but there have also been a few clinical trials in humans. In other chapters, we have already discussed some new research which might be considered gene therapy. For example, cytokine and other genes are being inserted into tumor cells to make vaccines. We have mentioned the possibility of inserting drug resistance genes into bone marrow and other target cells for drugs, to be able to give higher doses of cancer drugs without toxic side effects. But there are more exciting possibilities. Genes have already been put into tumor cells to make them sensitive to drugs which do not damage normal cells. Ultimately, researchers hope to even inactivate oncogenes and reactivate tumor suppressor genes in cancer cells.

Gene marker studies in humans

The first human cancer gene therapy experiments, however, were nothing grandiose: they were simply "gene marker" studies. In these studies, a gene is inserted into patients' cells which are scheduled to be returned to the body. This gene is not designed to cure anything; it is simply a tag for cells (it's as if researchers had painted a cell green or red to be able to identify it again in a crowd). For example, one gene marker study tracked "tumor infiltrating lymphocytes" (TILs), lymphocytes which were removed from the cancer and stimulated, then returned to the body in the hope that they would attack the cancer with increased force (Hermann, 1995). In this study, the TILs were marked with a gene to see whether they actually made it back to the cancer (They did.) Gene marker studies do not cure the cancer. What they are (besides interesting studies in their own right) is a way to test gene therapy and make sure that it is safe in humans. Gene marker studies have quieted some of the fears about the safety of gene therapy (Hermann, 1995).

Suicide genes

Researchers want to do more, however, than simply mark cells with genes; they want to cure cancer. One of the more interesting and practical ideas has been to put genes into cancer cells which will make the cancer cells very sensitive to ordinary, fairly nontoxic drugs. Sometimes, these genes are called "suicide genes"; the cells that pick them up are doing a suicidally dangerous thing. There are a number of different suicide genes. One of the most promising may be a virus enzyme called thymidine kinases.

Thymidine kinases (TK) converts Ganciclovir (a drug used to treat virus infections) from a nontoxic compound into a very toxic poison. In recent experiments, investigators put the *TK* gene into brain cancers in rats (Davis, 1996). After cancer cells had incorporated the *TK* gene, the rats were given Ganciclovir. Cancer cells which carried the *TK* gene were killed by Ganciclovir (Figure 27.1). Normal cells were not. Researchers saw complete regression in 11 of 14 tumors, with no damage to nearby normal tissues. One of the interesting things about this treatment is that tumors regressed when as few as one out of every ten cancer cells had incorporated the *TK* gene (Hermann, 1995; Davis, 1996). Researchers don't exactly know how this happened; they do, however, know that the effect depended on "gap junctions," connections between neighboring cells which allow some chemicals and communications to pass between the cells. *TK* and Ganciclovir have also been promising in mice with oral (mouth) cancer, colon cancer and a type of leukemia (Davis, 1996).

Tests of thymidine kinases in humans have already begun. In one small study, nine patients with advanced ovarian cancer received the TK gene: one of those nine patients had a complete remission (Davis, 1996). An ongoing trial is testing whether thymidine kinases can kill cancer cells in human brain tumors (Davis, 1996). In this study, cells which make thymidine kinases were put directly into brain tumors, in the hopes that the thymidine kinases they made would kill the cancer cells when they were exposed to Ganciclovir. No results have yet been published from this study, but early reports indicate that some patients have responded.

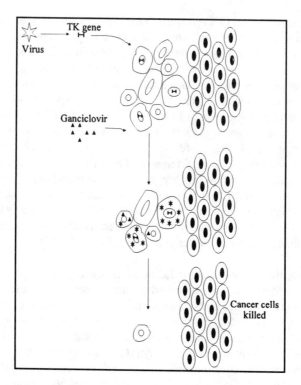

Figure 27.1. TK genes from a virus can make cancer cells susceptible to killing by Ganciclovir.

The previous TK gene experiments have all, however, had one problem common to gene therapy: getting the genes into the right cells. The solution, in most of these experiments, was to place the gene (in its virus or liposomes) near the cancer cells. A new refinement has, however, been able to send the TK suicide gene directly to any selected cell, even if it the gene is simply injected into the body (Davis, 1996). In this new technique, the TK gene was again put into viruses - but, this time, the gene could be turned on only by proteins found in cancer cells. In the first experiments, the gene was designed to work only in melanocytes and in their cancerous progeny, melanomas. Even if the TK gene accidentally got into other cells, it could not be turned on. When this form of the TK gene was injected into mice with metastatic melanoma, the number of metastasis dropped dramatically. Other TK genes have been designed to work only in stomach cancers or in liver cancers (Davis, 1996).

Replacing defective tumor suppressor genes

A more ambitious goal is to try to change the genes involved in cancers, including tumor suppressor genes. Recent advances have emphasized how widespread tumor suppressor gene mutations are in cancers. Replacing these defective genes is probably on every cancer researcher's wish list - and the gene at the top of those lists is probably *p53*. In fact, early gene therapy with *p53* has already been tried. In the laboratory, inserting the *p53* gene into cancer cells can trigger apoptosis in cells from a wide variety of cancers (Davis, 1996; Barinaga, 1997b) The *p53* gene (carried in liposomes) has also been safely delivered to lung cancers in mice; these tumors may regress and go into remission for a time (Davis, 1996; Wills, 1994). *P53* carrying viruses are also being tested in human safety trials (Barinaga, 1997b). No side effects have yet been seen and, in preliminary reports, researchers say that some tumors have regressed or stopped growing.

These studies are, of course, only a start. Although the preclinical trials have been somewhat successful, it seems unlikely that gene therapy for tumor suppressor genes will be completely effective until the genes can be delivered into a greater percentage of the tumor cells. It is also not yet useful for metastatic cancer, since the genes must be injected directly into tumors (Barinaga, 1997b). Yet it is encouraging to see how far tumor suppressor gene therapy has come. Not so long ago, we didn't even know p53 existed; today, it is already being tested for safety in cancer patients.

Inactivating oncogenes

The flip side of the coin to turning on tumor suppressor genes is, of course, turning off oncogenes. Inactivating oncogenes is rather different from the types of gene therapy we have mentioned so far. When we are dealing with tumor suppressor genes, suicide genes, or cytokines, the idea is to put a new gene into a cell- something that genetic researchers have considerable experience with. Turning off a gene, however, is not as straightforward. Rarely is it the case that we could simply put another gene inside the cell, which could turn the defective gene off. Instead, the problem gene must be turned off more directly.

There are several ways to inactivate genes. Mostly, they involve preventing the formation of messenger RNA (mRNA) from the gene, or destroying the mRNA once it is made. If you recall from chapter 2, active genes make messenger RNA, the molecule that eventually gets translated into protein. Get rid of the messenger RNA from a particular gene, and no protein is made. The gene itself becomes harmless and silent. The trick is, of course, to get rid of the oncogene's messenger RNAs without damaging other messenger RNAs in the cell. (It might make matters worse if you inactivated the oncogene you were targeting, but simultaneously destroyed other mRNAs which control cell growth). Three common methods use antisense molecules, ribozymes, and "triple-helix forming oligo-DNA" (Hermann, 1995).

Antisense molecules

Using an antisense molecule is one of the oldest methods to destroy specific pieces of messenger RNA. An antisense molecule is a small piece of DNA (with only one strand) or RNA, often chemically modified to make it last longer in a cell. Its bases are designed to attach only to messenger RNAs from a specific gene, and not to other messenger RNAs.

Antisense molecules (Figure 27.2) block their attached mRNA from ever being translated into protein (Hermann, 1995). Their presence on mRNA also attracts cutting enzymes, which cut this peculiar two-stranded mRNA into useless pieces (Roush, 1997a).

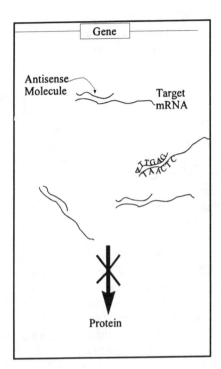

Figure 27.2 Antisense molecules attach to messenger RNA from a specific gene and prevent it from being translated into protein.

Although researchers have tried to use antisense molecules to treat various diseases, including cancer, these experiments have been plagued with problems. Antisense molecules don't always work as planned. For example, in one early study of an autoimmune disease called lupus erythematosus, antisense molecules were designed to turn off the overactive immune response causing the disease. Instead, they actually turned the activity up higher (Roush, 1997a). In other studies, the antisense molecules seemed to work - but antisense molecules made of random nonsensical bases, which were not designed to attach to the target mRNAs, seemed to work almost as well! (Roush, 1997a) Now it seems that researchers have worked out some of these problems (which may have been due to the way the antisense molecules were constructed) and they hope that a new generation of antisense drugs may work a bit better (Roush, 1997a).

A diverse group of these new antisense molecules have been tried in laboratory animals and humans. In small human (phase I) safety trials reported at the American Society of Clinical Oncology meeting in 1997, antisense molecules appeared to be safe in human patients with ovarian cancer (Roush, 1997a). In fact, the antisense drugs were able to stop the growth of ovarian tumors in three of 17 patients. An antisense molecule has also been made for the *Ras* oncogene and may soon be tested in clinical trials in humans (Hermann, 1995). Some researchers are attempting to suppress the oncogene *bcl-2*, which prevents apoptosis, using antisense DNA (Barinaga, 1997b). In this trial, one partial remission and one complete remission were seen among nine patients with lymphoma. Promising preclinical trials in breast cancers in laboratory animals, using antisense molecules for the oncogene *fos*, have also been reported (Arteaga, 1996).

Still, antisense molecules have a long way to go before they are a practical treatment for cancer. One problem is the expense. Because some antisense molecules simply attach more strongly to some mRNAs than others, researchers must screen an estimated 30 to 40 molecules to find one that works well (Roush, 1997a). At $2000 for a gram of each one, that can get pretty expensive! Other problems include getting the antisense molecules into the nuclei of the right cells, as well as continuing doubts that they are actually working as they are expected to work, and not by some completely unexpected means (which might later result in some unexpected side effects) (Roush, 1997a).

Ribozymes and triple helix forming oligo DNAs

Ribozymes are unusual pieces of RNA which can actually act as enzymes. (They're odd little creatures that are used by the cell to modify bits of RNA in the cell's nucleus.) Artificial ribozymes can be made which attach to specific mRNAs, just as antisense RNAs do. But, in this case, the ribozymes are a bit more direct about it: they actually cut up the mRNA they've attached themselves to and destroy it.

Triple helix forming oligo DNAs are little bits of DNA which can attach directly to the malfunctioning gene and turn it off. Like the antisense molecules, they are small, single stranded pieces of DNA designed to attach to a specific sequence. But these molecules are pretty special; they can actually attach to a double stranded piece of DNA and convert it into a triple strand. The enzymes which make messenger RNAs from DNA are not capable of dealing with triple stranded DNA (they are used to the usual double stranded form). So they stop (presumably quite puzzled!) and leave that gene strictly alone. No mRNA is made at all and the gene becomes harmless.

Of these three techniques for turning off genes, the triple helix forming oligo DNAs are the least developed for cancer treatment. They have not yet been used inside a living organism (Hermann, 1995). Ribozymes have, however, been tested on a limited scale, with limited success (Hermann, 1995; Davis, 1996).

Cancer gene therapy in humans: where are we?

As we have seen, tests of cancer gene therapy in humans are only beginning (with the exception of gene modified vaccines). Researchers are slowly moving beyond gene marker studies into gene therapy designed to cure. At the moment, suicide genes seem to show the most immediate promise. Although they share some problems common to gene therapy, such as ensuring accurate delivery to cells and preventing damage to other genes, they do not face some of the other obstacles. Tumor suppressor genes will, seemingly, only be fully effective once they can be delivered to a large percentage of the cells in a tumor. Oncogene suppression shares the same problem, but also faces some unusual technical problems of its own. It seems quite likely that these problems will eventually be overcome. Nevertheless, gene therapy is still a science in its infancy: it shows great potential, but has yet to grow up and fulfill that promise.

Chapter 28

Learning to prevent cancer

No matter how sophisticated or advanced they are, cancer treatments are often uncomfortable, usually unpleasant - and never quite certain. In spite of all of the new advances, there are no miracle cures. It might be sobering to realize that the death rate from many metastatic cancers of has not decreased over the last 25 years (Hong, 1997). Once the cancer has reached a certain stage, it becomes very, very difficult to stop. At the moment, the best chance for a cancer cure is simply to catch it very early. Numerous research efforts are aimed at finding new methods to detect cancers early. Others, however, are attempting to prevent cancers from ever developing.

A certain amount of cancer prevention rests on individual choices. Choosing not to smoke can vastly reduce the risk of lung cancer. Wearing sun screen consistently can greatly reduce the risk of skin cancer. Making dietary choices that are high in antioxidant-containing vegetables and relatively low in fat, can reduce the risk of other cancers. Limiting sexual partners and practicing safe sex can reduce the risk of infection with the human papillomaviruses, and the risk of cervical cancer. Handling radiation carefully, limiting pollutants, and avoiding known carcinogens can also aid in cancer prevention.

Nevertheless, it seems very unlikely that cancer will ever be completely preventable through lifestyle choices. We cannot eliminate the risk of cancer from cosmic rays, from the estimated 50 percent of natural carcinogens in our food, or from genetic risk factors. Nor does it seem likely that human beings will always be willing to do the safest thing for them; a small increase in the risk of cancer 20 or 30 years away doesn't often outweigh the satisfaction of a charcoal broiled hamburger and fries right now. Some choices are just easier than others! Cancer is likely to be with us, no matter how careful or prudent our society becomes. There is, however, great hope in the early detection of abnormal cells and early interventions to prevent those cells from turning into actual cancers.

Chemoprevention

Chemoprevention is the prevention of cancer with drugs. The ultimate goal of chemoprevention is to prevent abnormal cells from ever forming. At the moment, however, a more practical goal is the reversal or destruction of early cancers, at the stage where the cells are abnormal but have not yet become cancerous. Such groups of abnormal cells are called premalignant lesions. Premalignant lesions are, in a sense, halfway between normal cells and cancer cells. At this stage, they are more likely to respond to normal cell controls than they will be later.

Many chemoprevention drugs may be useful both for reversing premalignant lesions and for preventing cancer. Generally, new drugs are tested first for their effectiveness against premalignant lesions (or very early cancers). Later, if they show promise, they may be tested for their ability to prevent cancer in the general population. This is done for logistical reasons. Testing a drug as a preventative must be done on extremely large numbers of people, for several years at least, to see a decrease in the number of cases of cancer. There are simply too few cases of cancer expected in any small group of people to be able to detect a significant difference with or without the drug. People who already have premalignant lesions, however, already have a much higher chance of getting cancer; if the drug is effective, a difference can be seen in a much smaller group of people. The science of chemoprevention is still in its infancy, yet there are already signs of hope for specific cancers.

Hormone inhibitors in breast and prostate cancers

One of the more active areas in chemoprevention is the prevention of breast and prostate cancers with drugs that suppress hormones.

Breast cancers and estrogen inhibitors

Estrogen inhibitors have been quite promising as preventatives for breast cancer. As mentioned previously (chapter 15), however, estrogen has many functions in the body and many of them are beneficial. Inhibiting all of estrogen's effects would increase the risk of heart disease, osteoporosis, and possibly other diseases. What physicians need is a drug which could inhibit the effects of estrogen on the breast, without affecting its actions on other organs. Tamoxifen comes close. It acts like estrogen on the heart and bone, but inhibits estrogen in the breast. Unfortunately, Tamoxifen acts like estrogen in the uterus, as well, and may increase the risk of cancers of the uterus (Kennemans, 1996; Wilking, 1997).

In spite of this drawback, Tamoxifen has been tested as a cancer preventative in animals and in humans at high risk for breast cancer. In one study, Tamoxifen was given to women who had survived one breast cancer and had a high risk of developing a second tumor (Hong, 1997). The women who took Tamoxifen had 40 percent fewer new tumors than those who did not. Based on these promising results, Tamoxifen was recently tested in 13,000 healthy women (Hong, 1997). Some of the participants were older women, who qualified for the trial simply on the basis of age. Younger women who had a high risk for breast cancer could also enroll. This trial was stopped prematurely when researchers found that Tamoxifen was clearly beneficial in breast cancer prevention (Marshall, 1998). Women who took Tamoxifen had 45 percent fewer cases of breast cancer than women who did not. These women also had fewer bone fractures. There were, however, drawbacks to taking Tamoxifen. The risk of cancer of the uterus was twice as high in women getting Tamoxifen, and the risk of developing blood clots in the lung was three times as high. These risks only showed up in the older women in the study; women who started taking Tamoxifen when they were under 50 did not seem to have the same side effects.

Newer drugs, such as Raloxifene and LY353381, may come closer to the ideal breast cancer preventative (Hong, 1997). Neither promotes cancer of the uterus, and both mimic estrogen in bone and heart. LY353381 has been shown to prevent breast cancer in animals. The advantage of Raloxifene is that it is already used to prevent osteoporosis in women and is known to be safe in humans.

Prostate cancer and anti-androgens

Just as breast cancer can be driven by estrogens, prostate cancer is driven by androgens. In early cases of prostate cancer, depriving the tumor of testosterone may be able to stop or even reverse its growth. Drugs such as Finasteride, Flutamide, goserelin and leuprorelin have been used for the treatment of early cases of prostate cancers (chapter 15). Of these, Finasteride seems to be most promising for cancer prevention. It is an androgen inhibitor which lowers the concentration of active androgens by preventing the conversion of testosterone to the more active dihydrotestosterone (Hong, 1997). Finasteride does not completely suppress testosterone. It may, however, reduce it enough to lower the risk of prostate cancer, without the side effects expected from a severe reduction in testosterone levels. Over 18,000 men (aged 55 and over) are currently enrolled in a clinical trial to test Finasteride for the prevention of prostate cancer (Hong, 1997). The results of this study are expected in 5 or 6 years.

Vitamins in cancer prevention

Diets high in certain fruits and vegetables can reduce the risk of some cancers (Sankaranaryanan, 1996; Gaziano, 1996). Researchers suspect that the active ingredients in these foods might be vitamins. Vitamins, and relatives of vitamins, are attractive as cancer preventatives. Although some of them can be very dangerous when they are taken in large doses, others seem to be relatively harmless. Many vitamins are antioxidants. Antioxidants are chemicals which can neutralize free radicals, those dangerous molecules with an extra electron. Free radicals form in every cell, as a consequence of normal cell processes. They are also produced by exposure to sunlight and cigarette smoke, as well as other chemicals (Starr, 1997). The antioxidants essentially "mop up" the free radicals soon after they are formed and before they get a chance to do damage. Antioxidants are thought to be important in the prevention of cancer (Gaziano, 1996).

Beta carotene - cancer preventative gone bad?

Beta carotene and other carotenoids are found in yellow and leafy green vegetables and are converted into vitamin A in the body (Berkow, 1992). In early laboratory studies and small clinical trials, beta carotene seemed to be quite promising as a cancer preventative. As a result, some large clinical trials were begun, to fully evaluate beta carotene. In these trials, several thousand people took beta carotene pills to supplement their normal diets. Researchers followed these people for years, hoping to find that people who took the beta carotene supplements had fewer cases of cancer (and heart disease) than those who did not. Unfortunately, these trials only proved that beta carotene pills were poor cancer preventatives and even potentially dangerous.

The first trial, a study in Finland of 29,000 male smokers, startled researchers with some very unexpected results: not only did beta carotene supplements not prevent cancer, but they actually seemed to increase the risk of lung cancer in some people (Peterson, 1996; Albanes, 1995). Those men who took beta carotene supplements and either smoked or were exposed to high levels of asbestos had a 28 percent higher risk of lung cancer than those who did not take the supplements (Peterson, 1996). Beta carotene supplements also slightly increased the risk of prostate and stomach cancers (Albanes, 1995). As soon as these results became apparent, this trial was stopped early (Peterson, 1996). Beta carotene's reputation was further tarnished in trials sponsored by National Cancer Institute (Peterson, 1996). More than 22,000 people participated in this study, which found neither a risk nor a benefit to taking beta carotene for cancer prevention. In the National Cancer Institute trials, cancer risks did not increase in smokers. Only 11 percent of the participants in this trial were, however, smokers; some researchers speculate that there may have been too few smokers to see a subtle increase in the risks of lung cancer.

The U.S. Government has issued a statement that beta carotene supplements do not protect against cancer and may increase the risk of lung cancer in smokers (Santamaria, 1996). And researchers are scratching their heads like the rest of us, trying to figure it all out. One odd result from the Finnish study was that men who had higher beta carotene (and vitamin E) levels in the blood at the beginning of the study did, in fact, have a decreased risk of lung cancer (Albanes, 1995). It may be that beta carotene found in foods may be different from beta carotene found in a pill. Another possibility is that the high beta carotene levels may just be a coincidence; perhaps something else is present in foods high in beta carotene which prevents cancer. Some researchers even dispute the findings of these large studies, pointing out their own studies in cancer prevention in mice (Santamaria, 1996). At the moment, there seems to be no dispute about the benefits of eating vegetables to prevent cancer. But beta carotene pills seem to have become pointless, and possibly even dangerous.

Other antioxidants - Vitamins C and E

Vitamins C (ascorbic acid) and E (alpha tocopherol) are also being investigated as cancer preventatives. Eating foods which are high in these vitamins seems to decrease the risk of some forms of cancer. (Albanes, 1995; National Cancer Institute, 1997b). Both vitamins appear to be able to reduce DNA damage by some chemicals or x-rays, and increase the survival of cells in the laboratory (Sweetman, 1997). Vitamin C, for example, can be protective when cells are exposed to damaging doses of x-rays, and vitamin E has been able to protect cells from hydrogen peroxide, an antiseptic which kills bacteria by forming free radicals (Sweetman, 1997).

The National Cancer Institute is currently sponsoring studies to determine whether cancer can be prevented by vitamin C (National Cancer Institute, 1997b). Vitamin E (alpha tocopherol) has already been tested for cancer prevention in a large study of over 29,000 male smokers (together with vitamin A, whose results are described above). Vitamin E, unlike beta carotene in the same study, did actually seem to suppress the growth of some cancers (Albanes, 1995). Prostate and colon cancers occurred less often in those taking vitamin E supplements than those not taking them. Unfortunately, the supplements also seemed to increase the risk of cancers of the stomach. The message seems to be equivocal: eating foods high in vitamin E seems to be beneficial, but vitamin E pills may increase the risk of some forms of cancer while decreasing others.

Others vitamins, or their byproducts, may regulate normal cell development. Of these, the retinoids, chemicals which are normally made from vitamin A in the body, seem to be one of the most promising.

Lung cancers and other uses of the retinoids

Lung cancer is one of the deadliest of all cancers. It tends to remain undetected until it is widespread, and the cancers can develop quickly. Smokers often develop premalignant lesions throughout the lung. One hope for reversing these lesions is the retinoids. The retinoids stimulate the differentiation of cells and simultaneously decrease their potential for cell division (Hong, 1997). Retinoids have been able to reverse some premalignant lesions (Hong, 1997; Sankaranaryanan, 1996). Several retinoids have also been tested in clinical trials as cancer preventatives for patients who have had lung cancers. So far they have not been consistently effective in returning precancerous changes in the lungs and airways to normal (Sankaranaryanan, 1996). Currently, a combination of a retinoid and vitamin E is being tested in humans with premalignant lesions in the lungs (Hong, 1997).

Retinoids may also be useful for other cancers. Some breast cancer cells, for example, may also remain responsive to the retinoids. A retinoid (Fentretinate) in combination with Tamoxifen has also been very effective in preventing experimental breast cancer in animals, and is now in clinical trials with women (Hong, 1997; Sankaranaryanan, 1996). Retinoids have also been able to prevent the development of some skin cancers. One synthetic retinoid was given to patients who had already had one squamous cell carcinoma (a type of skin cancer) (Sankaranaryanan, 1996). During the following year, 24% percent of patients who did not get the retinoid developed a second squamous cell carcinoma; however, only four percent of patients who were treated with retinoic acid developed a second tumor. Unfortunately, the retinoids affect the development of many lining tissues; the side effects of retinoid treatment include dry skin, conjunctivitis (red and irritated eyes), and a potentially dangerous elevation in fats in the blood (Hong, 1997). New retinoids are being developed which are expected to have fewer side effects.

Colon cancer and COX-2 inhibitors

An enzyme known as cyclooxygenase 2 (COX-2) seems to be important in the early stages of colon cancer. The importance of COX-2 was discovered in mice with defects in the *APC* gene (Hong, 1997). Both humans and mice with defective *APC* genes tend to develop large numbers of polyps, small growths, in their intestines. These polyps are not dangerous in themselves; however, each polyp has the potential to develop into colon cancer. When researchers looked at polyps in the mice, they found excessive levels of the COX-2 enzyme. Mice with damage to both their *APC* genes and their *COX-2* genes, however, had far fewer polyps than mice with only *APC* defects. Somehow, the absence of COX-2 prevented the polyps from forming. (Some researchers think that COX-2 may prevent apoptosis in some cancer cells.) It turned out that human colon cancers also had high levels of COX-2. It seemed logical to see if treatments which inhibit COX-2 could prevent polyps from forming.

One cyclooxygenase inhibiting drug, Sulindac, has been used to inhibit the formation of polyps in humans (Hong, 1997). Unfortunately, the side effects of Sulindac make it useless as a nontoxic preventative for polyps. Researchers hope to find a drug which can safely inhibit COX-2 without side effects. Some new drugs have been developed, and one has been tested in mice. A compound called MF-tricyclic has been given to mice with defective *APC* genes without ill effects (Hong, 1997). These mice developed fewer polyps than their litter mates which were not treated with MF-tricyclic. It remains to be seen if MF-tricyclic or similar drugs will be safe, non-toxic and effective in humans.

Vaccination

Chemoprevention seems to hold a good deal of promise for cancer prevention, with the gradual development of newer and more specific drugs. There is, however, another possibility. Boosting the natural defenses of the body with vaccination may be able to prevent some types of cancer. The most obvious cases for vaccination are the cancers which are associated with viruses, such as cervical cancers or some leukemias. If infection with the virus can be prevented, then risk of the cancer should be reduced. For example, vaccination with peptides from a virus associated with cervical cancer can give mice immunity from some cervical tumors (Melief, 1996). A vaccine for the Epstein-Barr virus has also been able to protect animals against the lymphomas associated with this virus (Rickinson, 1995). Phase I clinical trials of this vaccine in humans are being planned (Rickinson, 1995).

Most cancers are not, however, associated with particular viruses. Vaccines against such cancers face some challenging obstacles.   In animal studies, it can be easier to prevent the establishment of cancers than to treat existing ones. In these experiments, however, investigators deliberately inject the mice with cancer cells; they know what antigens to expect on those cancers. The biggest obstacle to developing human anti-cancer vaccines is that the antigens on spontaneously developing human tumors can be unpredictable. This is not a small challenge, but the rewards are great. If this obstacle can be overcome, then, perhaps someday, vaccines against cancers might become as common as vaccines against infections.

Epilogue

Writing about cancer research has been a bit like wrestling with an octopus; you get one part under control and the rest squirms away from you. The field has exploded recently, with new developments in every direction: chemotherapy, hyperthermia, immune treatments, phototherapy, hormone and growth factor suppression, vitamin derivatives, gene therapy, blood vessel inhibition, apoptosis... and all of them constantly advancing! There are even new developments in those old standbys, radiation therapy and surgery. Undoubtedly, in the confusion, I have missed some valuable new research that should have been included.

But there is another aspect of cancer treatment that, I think, needs to be addressed in a final note. Cruise the Internet someday in your spare time, and I can guarantee that you will encounter some very bizarre cancer treatments. Some of them will sound plausible, if you don't remember much about biology. Others will startle you by their lack of common sense. It seems that, even all these years after the "traveling salesman," there are people who will be happy to sell just about anything. So I'll end this book with a plea: when you encounter new treatments and new possibilities, keep an open mind--but, at the same time, be very, very skeptical. Check for scientific evidence, and talk to your doctor. Some useless treatments will do more harm to your wallet than your body. Others can be dangerous. Yet others may delay you from seeking conventional treatments and reduce the chance of a cure.

Some of you reading this book will encounter cancer in your own lives. Current statistics estimate that one out of every three people will get cancer during their lifetime (Kuby, 1997). Treatments may have changed by then, but the biology of the tumor won't. If you take just one bit of knowledge about cancer away, it should be this: every day, every month, every year gives the cancer time to grow and spread and become more dangerous. Caught early, many cancers can be cured. Caught late, very few can. The main enemy is time.

Appendix

References

Abbas, A.A., A.H. Lichtman, and J.S. Pober. 1994. Cellular and molecular immunology, 2nd Ed. W.B. Saunders Co., Philadelphia.

Abdel-Wahab, Z., C. Weltz, D. Hester, N. Pickett, C. Vervaert, J.R. Barber, D. Jolly, and H.F. Siegler. 1997. A phase I clinical trial of immunotherapy with interferon-gamma gene-modified autologous melanoma cells: monitoring the humoral immune response. *Cancer* **80**:401-412.

Adams, A. 1998. 10-gallon molecule stomps tumors. *Science* **279**:1307-1308.

Ahmed, R. And D. Gray. 1996. Immunologic memory and protective immunity: understanding their relation. *Science* **272**:54-60.

Aisner, J. and H. Cortes-Funes. 1997. Paclitaxel in head and neck and other cancers: future prospects. *Semin. Oncol.* **24**:S2-113-S2-115.

Albanes, D., O.P. Heinonen, J.K. Huttunen, P.R. Taylor, J. Virtamo, B.K. Edwards, J. Haapakoski, M. Rautalahti, A.M. Hartman, J. Palmgren, et. al. 1995. Effects of alpha-tocopherol and beta-carotene supplements on cancer incidence in the Alpha-Tocopherol-Beta-Carotene Cancer Prevention Study. *Am. J. Clin. Nutr.* **62 (6 Suppl)**:1427S-1430S.

Altaner, C. 1995. Gene therapy for cancer (present status). *Neoplasma* **42**:209-213.

American Cancer Society. 1998. Who survives breast cancer? American Cancer Society [Online]. Available: http://www.cancer.org/statistics/97bcff.survive.html. [5 Feb 1998]

Ames, B.N. and L. Swirsky Gold. 1990 Chemical carcinogenesis: too many rodent carcinogens. *Proc. Natl. Acad. Sci. USA* **87**:7772-7776.

Anon. 1996. Gene modulates prostate cancer risk. *Science* **272**:1271.

Anon. 1997. Anticancer Compound Synthesized. *Science* **278**:1571.

Anon. 1998a. Dendritic cells offer potential treatment for cancer, HIV. The Scientist [Online]. Available: http://www.the-scientist.library.upenn.edu/yr1998/jan/research_ 980119.html. [19 Jan 1998].

Anon. 1998b. Pharmacology of Paclitaxel and Docetaxel. [Online]. Available: http://biotech.chem.indiana.edu/botany/tax.html [Mar 1998].

Arap, W., R. Pasqualini, and E. Ruoslahti. 1998. Cancer treatment by targeted drug delivery to tumor vasculature in a mouse model. Science 279:377-380.

Aziz, S.M., M.N. Gillespie, P.A. Crooks, S.F. Tofiq, C.P. Tsuboi, J.W. Olson, and M.P. Grosland. 1996. The potential of a novel polyamine transport inhibitor in cancer chemotherapy. J. Pharmacol. Exp. Ther. 278:185-192.

Azuma, A., H. Yagita, K. Okumura, S. Kudoh, and H. Niitani. 1994. Potentiation of long-term-cultured lymphokine-activated killer cell cytotoxicity against small-cell lung carcinoma by anti-CD3 x anti-(tumor-associated-antigen) bispecific antibody. Cancer Immunol. Immunother. 38:294-298.

Bacus, S.S., Y. Yarden, M.Oren, D.M. Chin, L. Lyass, C.R. Zelnick, A. Kazarov, W. Toyofuku, J. Gray-Bablin, R.R. Beerli, N.E. Hynes, M. Nikiforov, R. Haffner, A. Gudkov, and K. Keyomarsi. 1996. Neu differentiation factor (Heregulin) activates a p53-dependent pathway in cancer cells. Oncogene 12:2535-2547.

Barinaga, M. 1995. Two major signaling pathways meet at MAP-kinase. Science 269:1673.

Barinaga, M. 1996a. Forging a path to cell death. Science 273:735-736.

Barinaga, M. 1996b. Life-death balance within the cell. Science 274:724.

Barinaga, M. 1997a. Designing therapies that target blood vessels. Science 275:482-484.

Barinaga, M. 1997b. From bench top to bedside. Science 278:1036-1039.

Barinaga, M. 1997c. Molecules give new insights into deadliest brain cancers. Science 278:1226.

Barinaga, M. 1997d. The telomerase picture fills in. Science 276: 528-529.

Barinaga, M. 1998a. Peptide-guided cancer drugs show promise in mice. Science 279:323-324.

Barinaga, M. 1998b. Study suggests new way to gauge prostate cancer risk. *Science* **279**:475.

Baselga, J. and J. Mendelsohn. 1994. The epidermal growth factor as a target for therapy in breast carcinoma. *Breast Cancer Res. Treat.* **29**:127-138.

Baskar, S. 1996. Gene-modified tumor cells as cellular vaccine. *Cancer Immunol. Immunother.* **43**:165-173.

Bear, H.D., G.G. Hamad, and P.J. Kostuchenko. 1996. Biologic therapy of melanoma with cytokines and lymphocytes. *Semin. Surg. Oncol.* **12**:436-445.

Ben-Efraim, S. 1996. Cancer immunotherapy: hopes and pitfalls: a review. *Anticancer Res.* **16**:3235-3240.

Bender MedSystems. 1998. Tumor biology-p185HER-2. Bender Medsystems - Scientific Information [Online]. Available: http://www.bi-bioproducts.de/products/immunology/tumor_biology/tumor_biology_p185.shtml [Apr 1998].

Arioka, H. and N. Saijo. 1994. [Microtubules and antineoplastic drugs] *Gan To Kagaku Ryoho* **21**:583-590.

Benner, S.E., S.M. Lippman, and W.K. Hong. 1994. Retinoid chemoprevention of second primary tumors. *Semin. Hematol.* **31 (4 Suppl 5)**:26-30.

Berd, D., H.C. Maguire Jr., L.M. Schuchter, R. Hamilton, W.W. Hauck, T. Sato, and M.J. Mastrangelo. 1997. Autologous hapten-modified melanoma vaccine as postsurgical adjuvant treatment after resection of nodal metastases. *J. Clin. Oncol.* **15**:2359-2370.

Berkow, R. and A.J. Fletcher. 1992. The Merck manual of diagnosis and therapy, 17th Ed. Merck Research Laboratories, Rathway, N.J.

Bikfalvi, A. 1995. Significance of angiogenesis in tumour progression and metastasis. *Eur. J. Cancer* **31A**:1101-1104.

Bjarnason, G.A. 1995. Chronobiology Implications for cancer chemotherapy. *Acta Oncol.* **34**:615-624.

Blom, R., N. Palm, and E. Simonsen. 1996. Paclitaxel (Taxol) monotherapy in the treatment of progressive and recurrent ovarian carcinoma after platinum-based chemotherapy. *Acta Oncol.* **35**:733-736.

Blomqvist, C., T. Wiklund, M. Pajunen, M. Virolainen, and I Elomaa.1995. Oral Trofosfamide: an active drug in the treatment of soft-tissue sarcoma. *Cancer Chemother. Pharmacol.* **36**:263-265.

Boffetta, P. and J.M. Kaldor. 1994. Secondary malignancies following cancer chemotherapy. *Acta Oncol.* **33**:591-598.

Bolla, M., D. Gonzalez, P. Warde, J.B. Dubois, R.O. Mirimanoff, G. Storme, J. Bernier, A. Kuten, C. Sternberg, T. Gil, L. Collette and M. Pierart. 1997. Improved survival in patients with locally advanced prostate cancer treated with radiotherapy and goserelin. *N. Eng. J. Med.* **337**:295-300.

Boyle, R.W., J. Rousseau, S.V. Kudrevich, M. Obochi, and J.E. van Lier. 1996. Hexadecafluorinated zinc phthalocyanine: photodynamic properties against the EMT-6 tumour in mice and pharmacokinetics using 65Zn as a radiotracer. *Br. J. Cancer* **73**:49-53.

Brahme, A. 1996. Recent developments in radiation therapy planning and treatment optimization. *Australas. Phys. Eng. Sci. Med.* **19**:53-66.

Brodie, A.M. 1994. Aromatase inhibitors in the treatment of breast cancer. *J. Steroid Biochem. Mol. Biol.* **49**:281-287.

Brogden, R.N. and D. Faulds. 1995. Goserelin. A review of its pharmacodynamic and pharmacokinetic properties and therapeutic efficacy in prostate cancer. *Drugs Aging* **6**:324-343.

Brown, J.M. and A.J. Giaccia. 1994. Tumour hypoxia: the picture has changed in the 1990s. *Int. J. Radiat. Biol.* **65**:95-102.

Bruland, O.S. 1995. Cancer therapy with radiolabeled antibodies. An overview. *Acta Oncol.* **34**:1085-1094.

Brunda, M.J and M.K. Gately. 1995. Interleukin-12: potential role in cancer therapy. *Important Adv. Oncol.*:3-18.

Burner, N.G., R. Wurm, J. Nyman, and J.H. Peacock. 1996. Normal tissue radiosensitivity-- how important is it? *Clin. Oncol. (R. Coll. Radiol.)* **8**:25-34.

Buschbaum, D.J., D. Raben, M.A. Stackhouse, M.B. Khazaeli, B.E. Rogers, M.E.
    Rosenfeld, T. Liu, and D.T. Curiel. 1996. Approaches to enhance cancer
    radiotherapy employing gene transfer methods. *Gene Ther.* 3:1042-
    1068.

Carde, P., D.I. Rosenthal, C. Koprowski, R. Schea, J. Ruckle, R. Tishler, S.
    Young, R. Miller, M. Hohn, M.F. Renschler, and G. Roussy. 1997. A
    phase IB/II mutli-dose trial of gadolinium-Texaphyrin (Gd-Tex) as a
    radiosensitizer in patients with brain metastases: preliminary results
    (Abstract). *Proc. Annu. Meet. Am. Soc. Clin. Oncol.* 16:A1388.

Cersosimo, R.J. and D. Carr. 1996. Prostate cancer: current and evolving
    strategies. *Am. J. Health Syst. Pharm.* 53:381-396.

Chan, J.M., M.J. Stampfer, E. Giovannucci, P.H. Gann, J. Ma, P. Wilkinson, C.H.
    Hennekens, and M. Pollak. 1998. Plasma insulin-like growth factor-1
    and prostate cancer risk: a prospective study. *Science* 279: 563-566.

Chaux, P., M.S. Martin, and F. Martin. 1996. T-cell co-stimulation by the CD28
    ligand B7 is involved in the immune response leading to rejection of a
    spontaneously regressive tumor. *Int. J. Cancer* 66:244-248.

Cheville, N.F. 1983. Neoplasia. In Cell Pathology, 2nd Ed., 346-414. The Iowa
    State University Press, Ames, IA.

Chresta, C.M., E.L. Arriola, and J.A. Hickman. 1996. Apoptosis and cancer
    chemotherapy. *Behring Inst. Mitt.* (97):232-240.

Clarke, M.F., I.J. Apel, M.A. Benedict, P.G. Eipers, V. Sumatran, M. Gonzalez-
    Garcia, M. Doedens, N. Fukunaga, B. Davidson, J.E. Dick et. al. 1995.
    A recombinant bcl-xs adenovirus selectively induces apoptosis in cancer
    cells but not in normal bone marrow cells. *Proc. Natl. Acad. Sci. USA*
    92:11024-11028.

Clinton, G.M. and W. Hua. 1997. Estrogen action in human ovarian cancer.
    Crit. Rev. Oncol. Hematol. 25:1-9.

Conry, R.M., A.F. LoBuglio, and D.T. Curiel. 1996. Polynucleotide-mediated
    immunization therapy of cancer. *Semin. Oncol.* 23:135-147.

Conti, P., M. Reale, M. Nicolai, R.C. Barbacane, F.C. Placido, R. Iantorno, and R. Tenaglia. 1994. Bacillus Calmette-Guerin potentiates monocyte responses to lipopolysaccharide-induced tumor necrosis factor and interleukin-1, but not interleukin-6 in bladder cancer patients. *Cancer Immunol. Immunother.* **38**:365-371.

Coppola, G., M. Atlas-White, S. Katsahambas, J. Bertolini, M.T. Hearn, and J.R. Underwood. 1997. Effect of intraperitoneally, intravenously and intralesionally administered anti-beta-FGF antibodies on rat chondrosarcoma tumor vascularization and growth. *Anticancer Res.* **17**:2033-2039.

Cornic, M, A. Agadir, L. Degos, and C. Chomienne. 1994. Retinoids and differentiation treatment: a strategy for treatment in cancer. *Anticancer Res.* **14**:2339-2346.

Corvio, R. 1996. [Antioncogene p53 and apoptosis response: new hypotheses on the molecular bases of tumor resistance to radiotherapy] *Radiol. Med. (Torino)* **92**:298-302.

Coukell, A.J. and D. Faulds. 1997. Epirubicin. An updated review of its pharmacodynamic and pharmacokinetic properties and therapeutic efficacy in the management of breast cancer. *Drugs* **53**:453-482.

Craft, P.S. and A.L. Harris. 1994. Clinical prognostic significance of tumour angiogenesis. *Ann. Oncol.* **5**:305-311.

Cress, A.E. and W.S. Dalton. 1996. Multiple drug resistance and intermediate filaments. *Cancer Metastasis Rev.* **15**:499-506.

Crystal, R.G. 1995. Transfer of genes to humans: early lessons and obstacles to success. *Science* **270**:404-410.

De Boer, E.C., L. Somogyi, G.J. de Ruiter, T.M. Reijke, K.H. Kurth, and D.H. Schamhart. 1997. Role of interleukin-8 in inset of the immune response in intravesical BCG therapy for superficial bladder cancer. *Urol. Res.* **25**:31-34.

de Lange, T. 1998. Telomeres and senescence: ending the debate. *Science* **279**:334-335.

Dean, C., H. Modjtahedi, S. Eccles, G. Box, and J. Styles. 1994. Immunotherapy with antibodies to the EGF receptor. *Int. J. Cancer Suppl.* **8**:103-107.

Deehan, D.J., S.D. Heys, J. Ashby, and O. Eremin. 1995. Interleukin-2 (IL-2) augments host cellular immune reactivity in the perioperative period in patients with malignant disease. *Eur. J. Surg. Oncol.* **21**:16-22.

Dellian, M., C. Richert, F. Gamarra, and A.E. Goetz. 1996. Photodynamic eradication of amelanotic melanoma of the hamster with fast acting photosensitizers. *Int. J. Cancer* **65**:246-248.

Desai, K.N., H. Wei, and C. A. Lamartiere. 1996. The preventive and therapeutic potential of the squalene-containing compound, Roidex, on tumor promotion and regression. *Cancer Lett.* **101**:93-96.

Dickson, R.B., M.D. Johnson, M. Maemura, and J. Low. 1996. Anti-invasion drugs. *Breast Cancer Res. Treat.***38**:121-132.

Dillman, R.O. 1994a. Antibodies as cytotoxic therapy. *J. Clin. Oncol.* **12**:1497-515.

Dillman, R.O. 1994b. The clinical experience with interleukin-2 in cancer therapy. *Cancer Biother.* **9**:183-209.

Disis, M.L. and M.A. Cheever. 1997. HER-2/neu protein: a target for antigen-specific immunotherapy of human cancer. *Adv. Cancer Res.* **71**:343-371.

D'Hondt, V., Y. Humblet, T. Guillaume, S. Baatout, C. Chatelain, M. Berliere, F. Longueville, A.M. Feyens, J. deGreve, A. Van Oosterom et. al. 1995. Thrombopoietic effects and toxicity of interleukin-6 in patients with ovarian cancer before and after chemotherapy: a multicentric placebo-controlled, randomized phase IIb study. *Blood* **85**:2347-2353.

Eccles, S.A., G.M. Box, W.J. Court, E.A. Bone, W. Thomas, and P.D. Brown. 1996. Control of lymphatic and hematogenous metastasis of a rat mammary carcinoma by the matrix metalloproteinase inhibitor Batimastat (BB-94). *Cancer Res.* **56**:2815-2822.

Edwards, N. 1996. Taxol. School of Chemistry, University of Bristol [Online].Available: http://www.bris.ac.uk/Depts/Chemistry/ MOTMtaxol/taxol1.htm [May 1998].

Ehrenstein, D. 1998. Immortality gene discovered. *Science* **279**:177.

el-Deiry, W.S. 1997 Role of oncogenes in resistance and killing by cancer therapeutic agents. *Curr. Opin. Oncol.* **9**:79-87.

Elmajian, D.A., A.A. Agha, and D.J. Culkin. 1997. Metastatic prostate cancer: an update. *Hosp. Med.* **33**:48-52.

Engin, K. 1994a. Hyperthermia in cancer treatment (I). *Neoplasma* **41**:269-276. National Cancer Institute, 1997a

Engin, K. 1994b. Biological rationale for hyperthermia in cancer treatment (II). *Neoplasma* **41**:277-283.

Evensen, J.F. 1995. The use of porphyrins and non-ionizing radiation for treatment of cancer. *Acta Oncol.* **34**:1103-1110.

Ezaki, K. and M. Tsuzuki. 1997. Cytokine therapy for hematologic malignancies. *Gan To Kagaku Ryoho* **24 Suppl 1**:182-194.

Fearon, E. 1997. Human cancer syndromes: clues to the origin and nature of cancer. *Science* **278**:1043-1050.

Feldmann, H.J., M.H. Seegenschmiedt, and M. Molls. 1995. Hyperthermia-- its actual role in radiation oncology. Part III-Clinical rationale and results in deep seated tumors. *Strahlenther. Onkol.* **171**:251-264.

Fenner, F., P.A. Bachmann, E.P.J. Gibbs, F.A. Murphy, M.J. Studdert, and D.O. White. 1987. Mechanisms of viral tumorigenesis. In Veterinary virology, 217-236. Academic Press, San Diego, CA.

Fisher, G.A. and B.I. Sikic. 1995. Clinical studies with modulators of drug resistance. *Hematol. Oncol. Clin. North Am.* **9**:362-382.

Focan, C. 1995. Circadian rhythms and cancer chemotherapy. *Pharmac. Ther.* **67**:1-52.

Frankel, A.E., E.P. Tagge, and M.C. Willingham. 1995. Clinical trials of targeted toxins. *Semin. Cancer Biol.* **6**:307-317.

Friess, H., M. Gassmann, and M.W. Buchler. 1997. Adjuvant therapy of pancreatic cancer using monoclonal antibodies and immune response modifiers. *Int. J. Pancreatol.* **21**:43-52.

Furuya, Y.F., R. Berges, P. Lundmo, and J.T. Isaacs. 1994. Cell Proliferation, p53 gene expression and intracellular calcium in programmed cell death: prostate model. In Apoptosis II: the molecular basis of apoptosis in disease. Cold Spring Harbor Press. Plainview, NY.

Gallagher, R. 1997. Tagging T cells: TH1 or TH2? *Science* 275:1615.

Garbe, C. 1995. Perspectives of cytokine treatment in malignant skin tumors. *Recent Results Cancer Res.* 139:349-369.

Gattoni-Celli, S. and D.J. Cole. 1996. Melanoma-associated tumor antigens and their clinical relevance to immunotherapy. *Semin. Oncol.* 23:754-758.

Gaziano, J.M. and C.H. Hennekens. 1996. Update on dietary antioxidants and cancer. *Pathol. Biol. (Paris)* 44:42-45.

Glaspy, J. 1997. The impact of epoietin alpha on quality of life during cancer chemotherapy: a fresh look at an old problem. *Semin. Hematol.* 34:20-26.

Goa, K.L. and D. Faulds. 1994. Vinorelbine. A review of its pharmacological properties and clinical use in cancer chemotherapy. *Drugs Aging* 5:200-234.

Gonzalez Gonzalez D., J.D. van Dijk, and L.E. Blank. 1995. Radiotherapy and hyperthermia. *Eur. J. Cancer* 31A(7-8).

Green, D.R. 1997. A Myc-induced apoptosis pathway surfaces. *Science* 278:1246-1247

Grosland, M., B. Lum, J. Schimmelpfennig, J. Baker, and M. Doukas. 1996. Insights into mechanisms of Cisplatin resistance and potential for its clinical reversal. *Pharmacotherapy* 16:16-39.

Grunicke, H.H., K. Maly, F. Uberall, C. Schubert, E. Kindler, J. Stekar, and H. Brachwitz. 1996. Cellular signaling as a target in cancer chemotherapy. Phospholipid analogues as inhibitors of mitogenic sinal transduction. *Adv. Enzyme. Regul.* 36:385-407.

Gulati, S.C., R.M. Lemoli, T. Igarashi, and J. Atzpodien. 1994. Newer options for treating drug-resistant (MDR+) cancer cells using photoradiation therapy. *Leuk. Lymphoma* 12:427-433.

Gura, T. 1997a. Causing cancer by remote control? *Science* **276**:1788-1789.

Gura, T. 1997b. How TRAIL kills cancer cells but not normal cells. *Science* **277**:768.

Gura, T. 1997c. Systems for identifying new drugs are often faulty. *Science* **278**:1041-1042.

Gutterman, J.U. 1994. Cytokine therapeutics: lessons from interferon alpha. *Proc. Natl. Acad. Sci. USA* **91**: 1198-1205.

Hall, S.S. 1995. Monoclonal antibodies at age 20: promise at last? *Science* **270**:915-916.

Harris, A.L., H. Zhang, A. Moghaddam, S. Fox, P. Scott, A. Pattison, K. Gatter, I. Stratford, and R. Bicknell. 1996. Breast cancer angiogenesis - new approaches to therapy via antiangiogenesis, hypoxic activated drugs and vascular targeting. *Breast Cancer Res. Treat.* **38**:97-108.

Hartwell, L.H., P. Szankasi, C.J. Roberts, A.W. Murray, and S.H. Friend. 1997. Integrating genetic approaches into the discovery of anticancer drugs. *Science* **278**:1064-1068.

Hawkins, M.J., M.B. Atkins, J.P. Dutcher, R.I. Fisher, G.R. Weiss, K.A. Margolin, A.A. Rayner, M. Sznol, D.R. Parkinson, E. Paietta et. al. 1994. A phase II clinical trial of interleukin-2 and lymphokine-activated killer cells in advanced colorectal carcinoma. *I. Immunother.* **15**:74-78.

Hayes, R.L., M. Koslow, E.M. Hiesiger, K.B. Hymes, H.S. Hochster, E.J. Moore, D.M. Pierz, D.K. Chen, G.N. Budzilovich, and J. Ransohoff. 1995. Improved long term survival after intracavity interleukin-2 and lymphokine-activated killer cells for adults with recurrent malignant glioma. *Cancer* **76**:840-852.

Hermann F. 1995. Cancer gene therapy: principles, problems and perspectives. *J. Mol. Med.* **73**:157-163.

Hickman, J.A., C.S. Potten, A.J. Merritt, and T.C. Fisher. 1994. Apoptosis and cancer chemotherapy. *Philos. Trans. R . Soc. Lond. B. Biol. Sci.* **345**:319-325.

Holmes, F.A. 1996. Paclitaxel combination therapy in the treatment of metastatic breast cancer: a review. *Semin. Oncol.* **23(5 Suppl 11)**: 46-56.

Holtzman, N.A., P.D. Murphy, M.S. Watson, and P.A. Barr. 1997. Predictive genetic testing: from basic research to clinical practice. *Science* **278**:602-605.

Hong, W.K. and M.B. Sporn. 1997 Recent advances in chemoprevention of cancer. *Science* **278**:1073-1077.

Hahne, M., D. Rimoldi, M. Schroter, P. Romero, M. Schreier, L.E. French, P. Schneider, T. Bornand, A. Fontana, D. Lienard, J.-C. Cerrottini, and J. Tschopp. 1996. Melanoma cell expression of Fas (Apo-1/CD95) ligand: implications for tumor immune escape. *Science* **274**: 1363-1366.

Hortobagyi, G.N., R. Kilbourn and P. Weiden. 1998. A phase I multi-center study of E1A gene therapy for patients with epithelial ovarian cancer.Info.Resouce, Inc. [Online]. Available:

Hortobagyi, G.N. 1995. Management of breast cancer:status and future trends. *Semin. Oncol.* **22**:101-107.

Horwitz, S.B. 1994. Taxol (Paclitaxel): mechanisms of action. *Ann. Oncol.* **5 Suppl 6**:S3-6.

Hoskin, P.J., M.I. Saunders, H. Phillips, H. Cladd, M.E. Powell, K. Goodshild, M.R. Stratford, and A. Rojas. 1997. Carbogen and nicotinamide in the treatment of bladder cancer with radical radiotherapy. *Br. J. Cancer* **76**:260-263.

Huang, X., G. Molema, S. King, L. Watkins, T.S. Edgington, and P.E. Thorpe. 1997. Tumor infarction in mice by antibody-directed targeting of tissue factor to tumor vasculature. *Science* **275**:547-550.

Hung, M.C., A. Matin, Y. Zhang, X. Xing, F. Sorgi, L. Huang, and D. Yu. 1995. HER-2/neu-targeting gene therapy - a review. *Gene* **159**:65-71.

Husain, I., J.L. Mohler, H.F. Seigler, and J.M. Besterman. 1994. Elevation of topoisomerase I messenger RNA, protein, and catalytic activity in human tumors: demonstration of tumor-type specificity and implication for cancer chemotherapy.

Huyghenian, Y.A. 1997. Apoptosis and the dilemma of cancer chemotherapy. *Blood* **89**:1845-1853.

Itoh, K., A. Hayashi, Y. Toh, Y. Imai, A. Yamada, T. Nishida, and S. Shichijo. 1997. Development of cancer vaccine by tumor rejection antigens. *Int. Rev. Immunol.* **14**:153-171.

Jain, R.K. 1996. Delivery of molecular medicine to solid tumors. 1996. *Science* **271**:1079-1080.

Jendraschak, E. and E.H. Sage. 1996. Regulation of angiogenesis by SPARC and Angiostatin:implications for tumor cell biology. *Semin. Cancer Biol.* **7**:139-146.

Johnkoski, J.A., S.M. Peterson, R.J. Doerr, and S.A. Cohen. 1996. Levamisole regulates the proliferation of murine T cells through Kupffer-cell-derived cytokines. *Cancer Immunol. Immunother.* **43**: 299-306.

Kato, H. 1996. [History of photodynamic therapy--past, present and future]. *Gan To Kagaku Ryoho* **23**:8-15.

Kato, T., K. Sato, R. Sasaki, H. Kakinuma, and M. Moriyama. 1996. Targeted cancer chemotherapy with arterial microcapsule chemoembolization: review of 1013 patients. *Cancer Chemother. Pharmacol.* **37**:289-296.

Kennemans, P. 1996. Tamoxifen: alternative hormone replacement therapy with an anti-estrogen? *Eur. Menopause J.* **3**:5-6.

King, C.R., P.G. Kasprzyk, P.H. Fischer, R.E. Bird, and N.A. Turner. 1996. Preclinical testing of an anti-erbB-2 recombinant toxin. *Breast Cancer Res. Treat.* **38**:19-25.

Kirz, J. 1995. Remembering x-rays. *Science* **270**:934.

Klijn, J.G., B. Setyono-Han, H.J. Sander, S.W. Lamberts, F.H. de Jong, G.H. Deckers, and J.A. Foekens. 1994. Pre-clinical and clinical treatment of breast cancer with antiprogestins. *Hum. Reprod.* **9 Suppl 1**:181-189.

Korbelik, M., V.R. Naraparaju, and N. Yamamoto. 1997. Macrophage-directed immunotherapy as adjuvant to photodynamic therapy of cancer. *Br. J. Cancer* **75**:202-207.

Kreitman, R.J. and I. Pastan. 1994. Recombinant single-chain immunotoxins against T and B cell leukemias. *Leuk. Lymphoma* **13**: 1-10.

Krosl, G., M. Korbelik, and G.J. Dougherty. 1995. Induction of immune cell infiltration into murine SCCVII tumour by Photofrin-based photodynamic therapy. *Br. J. Cancer* 71:549-555.

Kuan, C.T. and I. Pastan. 1996 Improved antitumor activity of a recombinant anti-Lewis(y) immunotoxin not requiring proteolytic activation. *Proc. Natl. Acad. Sci. USA* 93:974-978.

Kuby, J. 1997. Immunology, 3rd Ed. W.H. Freeman and Co., New York.

Kuss, J.T., H.B. Muss, H. Hoen, and L.D. Case. 1997. Tamoxifen as initial endocrine therapy for metastatic breast cancer: long-term follow-up of two Piedmont Oncology Association (POA) trials. *Breast Cancer Res Treat.* 42:265-274.

Kuzel, T.M., H.H. Roenigk Jr., E. Samuelsen, J.J. Herrmann, A. Hurria, A.W. Rademaker, and S.T. Rosen. 1995. Effectiveness of interferon alfa-2a combined with phototherapy for mycosis fungoides and the Sezary syndrome. *J. Clin Oncol.* 13:257-263.

Lavelle, F., M.C. Bissery, C. Combeau, J.F. Riou, P. Vrignaud, and S. Andríe. 1995. Preclinical evaluation of Docetaxel (Taxotere). *Semin. Oncol.* 22:3-16.

Lavau, C. and A. Dejean. 1994. The t(15;17) translocation in acute promyelocytic leukemia. *Leukemia* 8 Suppl 2:S9-15.

Lawley, P.D. 1995. Alkylation of DNA and its aftermath. *Bioessays* 17:561-568.

Lee, D.J., M. Moini, J. Giuliano, and W.H. Westra. 1996. Hypoxic sensitizer and Cytotoxin for head and neck cancer. *Ann. Acad. Med. Singapore* 25:397-404.

Lee, L.F., C.C. Maly-Schuerer, A.K. Lofquist, C. van Haaften-Day, J.P. Ting, C.M. White, B.K. Martin, and J.S. Haskill. 1996. Taxol-dependent transcriptional activation of IL-8 expression in a subset of human ovarian cancer. *Cancer Res.* 56:1303-1308.

LeMaistre, C.F., C. Meneghetti, L. Howes, and C.K. Osborne. 1994. Targeting the EGF receptor in breast cancer treatment. *Breast Cancer Res. Treat.* 32:97-103.

Levine, A.J. 1997. p53, the cellular gatekeeper for growth and division. *Cell* **88**:323-331.

Lewis, C. 1994. A review of the use of chemoprotectants in cancer chemotherapy. *Drug Saf.* **11**:153-162.

Linehan, D.C., P.S. Goedegebuure, and T.J. Eberlein. 1996. Vaccine therapy for cancer. *Ann. Surg. Oncol.* **3**:219-228.

Lissoni, P., S. Barni, S. Meregalli, V. Fossati, M. Cazzaniga, D. Esposti, and G. Tancini. 1995. Modulation of cancer endocrine therapy by melatonin: a phase II study of Tamoxifen plus melatonin in metastatic breast cancer patients progressing under melatonin alone. *Br. J. Cancer* **71**:854-856.

Lissoni, P., G. Tancini, S. Barni, F. Paolorossi, A. Ardizzoia, A. Conti, and G. Maestroni. 1997. Treatment of cancer chemotherapy-induced toxicity with the pineal hormone melatonin. *Support. Care Cancer* **5**:126-129.

Look, K.Y. 1996. Rating the chemotherapy options for advanced uterine adenocarcinoma. *Medscape Women's Health* 1(11) [Online]. [Online] Available: http://www.medscape.com/Medscape/womens.health/1996/v01.n12/w17 [March 1996].

Look, A.T. 1997. Oncogenic transcription factors in the human acute leukemias. *Scinec* **278**:1059-1064.

Lum, B., J.T. Wieman, S. Taber, V. Fingar, D. Kessel, E Lowe, J. Engel , L. Parker, R. Miller, and M.F. Renschler. 1997.Pharmacodynamics of lutetium Texaphyrin (Lu-Tex) in a phase I trial of photodynamic therapy (PDT) of cancer (Abstract). *Proc. Annu. Meet. Am. Soc. Clin. Oncol.* **16**:A858

Maier-Lenz, H., J. Koetting, N. Onetto, N. Hollaender, T. Bauknecht, A. duBois, H.G. Meerpohl, K. Diergarten, and K. Mross. 1997. (Abstract). *Proc. Annu. Meet. Am. Assoc. Cancer Res.* **38**:A32.

Markman, M. and D.M. Peereboom. 1997. From serendipity to design: the evolution of drug development in oncology. *Cleve Clin. J. Med.* **64**:155-163.

Marshall, E. 1998. Tamoxifen. "A big deal" but a complex hand to play. *Science* **280**: 196.

Marx, J. 1994. How cells cycle toward cancer. *Science* **263**:319-321.

Marx, J. 1997. Possible function found for breast cancer genes. *Science* **276**: 531-532.

Masson, E. And W.C. Zamboni. 1997. Pharmacokinetic optimization of cancer chemotherapy. Effect on outcomes. *Clin. Pharmacokinet.* **32**:324-343.

Mastrangelo, M.J., H.C. Maguire, Jr., T. Sato, F.E. Nathan, and D. Berd. 1996. Active specific immunization in the treatment of patients with melanoma. *Semin. Oncol.* **23**:773-781.

Matzinger, P. 1998. The real function of the immune system. Tolerance and the four D's (danger, death, destruction and distress) [Online]. Available: Http://glamdring.ucsd.edu/others/aai/polly.html [Apr 1998].

McGinn, C.J., D.S. Shewach, and T.S. Lawrence. 1996. Radiosensitizing nucleosides. *J. Nat. Cancer Inst.* **88**:1193-1203.

Medscape. 1997. What are the roles of the taxanes in breast cancer? *J.M.C.C.* **4**:23-33 [Online] Available: http://www.Medscape.com/Moffitt/CancerControl/public/archive/1997/0403sup.toc.html [Feb 1997]

Melief, C.J.M., R. Offringa, R.E.M. Toes, and W.M. Kast. 1996. Peptide-based cancer vaccines. *Curr. Opin. Immunol.* **8**:651-657.

Mohanti, B.K., G.K. Rath, N. Anantha, V. Kannan, B.S. Das, B.A. Chandramouli, A.K. Banerjee, S. Das, A. Jena, R. Ravichandran, U.P. Sahi, R. Kumar, N. Kapoor, V.K. Kalia, B.S. Dwarakanath, and V. Jain. 1996. Improving cancer radiotherapy with 2-deoxy-D-glucose:phase I/II clinical trials on human cerebral gliomas. *Int. J. Radiat. Oncol. Biol. Phys.* **35**:103-111.

Momparler, R.L., J. Laliberte, N. Eliopoulos, C. Beausejour, and D. Cournoyer. 1996. Transfection of murine fibroblast cells with human cytidine deaminase cDNA confers resistance to cytosine arabinoside. *Anticancer Drugs* **7**:266-274.

Murdter, T.E., B. Sperker, K.T Kivisto, M. McClellan, P. Fritz, G. Friedel, A. Linder, K. Bosslet, H. Toomes, R. Dierkesmann, and H.K. Kroemer. 1997. Enhanced uptake of Doxorubicin into bronchial carcinoma: beta glucuronidase mediates release of Doxorubicin from a glucuronide prodrug (HMR 1826) at the tumor site. *Cancer Res.* **57**:2440-2445.

Musiani, P., A. Modesti, M. Giovarelli, F. Cavallo, M.P. Colombo, P.L. Lollini, and G. Forni. 1997. Cytokines, tumour-cell death and immnogenicity: a question of choice. *Immunol. Today* **18**:32-36.

Nagata, S. 1997. Apoptosis by death factor. *Cell* **88**:355-365.

Nardi, M., A. Aloe, S. De Marco, M. Atlante, A. Iacovellli, and F. Calabresi. 1996. Salvage therapy with Paclitaxel in advanced ovarian cancer: a phase II study (Abstract). *Proc. Am. Soc. Clin. Oncol.* **15**:A186.

National Cancer Institute. 1997a.Hyperthermia. CancerNet [Online]. Available: http://www.nci.nih.gov/clinpdq/therapy/Hyper thermia.html [Nov. 1997].

National Cancer Institute. 1997b. Vitamin C. CancerNet [Online]. Available: http://www.nci.nih.gov/clinpdq/therapy/VitaminC.html [Nov. 1997].

National Cancer Institute. 1998a. Autologous bone marrow transplantation in the treatment of breast cancer. CancerNet [Online]. Available: http://www.nci.nih.gov/clinpdq/therapy/Autologous_Bone_Marrow_ Transplantation_in_the Treatment_of_Breast_ Cancer.html [Jan 1998].

National Cancer Institute. 1998b. Lasers in cancer treatment. CancerNet [Online] Available: http://www.nci.nih.gov/clinpdq/therapy/Lasers_in_Cancer_ Treatment.html [Jan 1998].

National Cancer Institute. 1998c. Paclitaxel (Taxol, Registered trademark) and related anticancer drugs. CancerNet [Online]. Available: http://www.nci.nih.gov/clinpdq/therapy/Paclitaxel_(Taxol,Registered _Trademark)_and_Related_Anticancer_Drugs.html [Jan 1998].

National Cancer Institute. 1998d. PDQ Clinical trials information for physicians.CancerNet [Online]. Available: http://www.nci.nih.gov/clinpdq/therapy/PDQ_Clinical_ Trials_Information_for_Physicians/.html [Jan 1998].

National Cancer Institute. 1998e. Photodynamic therapy. CancerNet [Online]. Available: http://www.nci.nih.gov/clinpdq/therapy/Photodynamic Therapy.html [Jan 1998].

Nicolaou, K.C., N. Winssinger, J. Pastor, S. Ninkovic, F. Sarabia, Y. He, D. Vourloumis, Z. Yang, T. Li, P. Giannekakou, and E. Homel. 1997. Synthesis of epothilones A and B in solid and solution phase. *Nature* 387:268-272.

Niles, R.M. 1995. Use of vitamins A and D in chemoprevention and therpay of cancer: control of nuclear receptor expression and function. Vitamins, cancer and receptors. *Adv. Exp. Med. Biol.* 375:1-15.

Nomile, D. 1997. Heavy ions pack powerful punch. *Science* 278:1884.

Nooter, K. and G. Storer. 1996. Molecular mechanisms of multidrug resistance in cancer chemotherapy. *Pathol. Res. Pract.* 192:768-780.

Oka, S., T. Kubota, T. Takeuchi, and M. Kitajima. 1996. Potentiation of antitumor activity of mitomycin C by estradiol: studies of human breast carcinoma xenografts serially transplanted into nude mice. *J. Surg. Oncol.* 61:256-261.

Ono, K., S. Masunaga, K. Abuta, and M. Akaboshi. 1994. Middle dose rate irradiation in combination with carbogen inhalation selectively and more markedly increases the responses of SCCVII tumors. *Int. J. Radiat. Oncol. Biol. Phys.* 29:81-85.

O'Brien, C. 1996. New tumor suppressor found in pancreatic cancer. *Science* 271:294.

O'Reilly, S., M.J. Kennedy, E.K. Rowinsky, and R.C. Donehower. 1995. Vinorelbine and the topoisomerase I inhibitors: current and potential roles in breast cancer chemotherapy. *Breast Cancer Res. Treat.* 33:1-17.

O'Shaughnessy, J.A. and K.H. Cowan. 1995. Current status of Paclitaxel in the treatment of breast cancer. *Breast Cancer Res. Treat.* 33:27-37.

Pardoll, D. 1996. Releasing the brakes on antitumor immune responses. *Science* 271:1691.

Parhar, P., Y. Shi, M. Zou, N.D. Farid, P. Ernst, and S.T. Al-Sedairyl. 1995. Effects of cytokine-mediated modulation of nm23 expression on the invasion and metastatic behavior of B16F10 melanoma cells. *Int. J. Cancer* 60:204-210.

Parmiani, G., F. Arienti, J. Sule-Suso, C. Melani, M.P. Colombo, V. Ramakrishna, F. Belli, L. Mascheroni, L. Rivoltini, and N. Cascinelli. 1996. Cytokine-based gene therapy of human tumors. An overview. *Folia Biol. (Praha)* 42:305-309.

Patel, N.H. and M.L. Rosenburg. 1994. Multidrug resistance in cancer chemotherapy. *Invest. N. Drugs* 12:1-13.

Paulovich, A.G., D.P. Toczyski, and L.H. Hartwell. 1997. When checkpoints fail. *Cell* 88:315-321.

Peifer, M. 1997. B-catenin as oncogene:the smoking gun. *Science* 275:1752-1753.

Pennisi, E. 1996a. Drug's link to genes reveals estrogen's many sides. *Science* 273:1171.

Pennisi, E. 1996b. Gene linked to commonest cancer. Science 272:1583-1584.

Pennisi, E. 1996c. New gene forges link between fragile site and many cancers. *Science* 272:649.

Pennisi, E. 1996d. Teetering on the brink of danger. *Science* 271:1665-1667.

Pennisi, E. 1997. Superoxides relay ras protein's oncogenic message. *Science* 275:1567-1568.

Perera, F.P. 1997. Environment and cancer: who are susceptible? *Scinec* 278:1068-1073.

Peters, L.J. 1996. Radiation therapy tolerance limits. For one or for all? -- Janeway Lecture. *Cancer* 77:2379-2385.

Peterson, K. 1996. 'Natural' cancer prevention trial halted. *Science* 271:441.

Pharmacyclics. 1997. Lutetium Texaphyrin PCI-0123: a photosensitizer for photodynamic therapy of cancer. Pharmacyclics, Incorporated [Online]. Available: http://www.pcyc.com/Website/TechDocs/radiosen.htm #anchor88952 [March 1997].

Philip, P.A. and L. Flaherty. 1997. Treatment of malignant melanoma with interleukin-2. *Semin. Oncol.* 24:S32-8.

Pietersz, G.A. and K. Krauer. 1994. Antibody-targeted drugs for the therapy of cancer. *J. Drug Target.* 2:183-215.

Pietras, R.J., B.M. Fendly, V.R. Chazin, M.D. Pegram, S.B. Howell, and D.J. Slamon. 1994.

Plourde, P.V., M. Dyroff, M. Dowsett, L. Demers, R. Yates, and A. Webster. 1995. ARIMIDEX: a new oral, once-a-day aromatase inhibitor. *J. Steroid Biochem. Mol. Biol.* 53:175-179.

Ponder, B. Genetic testing for cancer risk. *Science* 278:1050-1054.

Pontiggia, P., F.C. Curto, A. Sabato, G.B. Rotella, and K. Alonso. 1995. Whole body hyperthermia in cancer therapy. Is metastatic breast cancer refractory to usual therapy curable? *Biomed. Pharmacother.* 49:79-82.

Pontiggia, P., G.B. Rotella, A. Sabato, and F.C. Curto. 1996. Therapeutic hyperthermia in cancer and AIDS: an updated survey. *J. Environ. Pathol. Toxicol. Oncol.* 15:289-297.

Prasad, K.N., C. Hernandez, J. Edwards-Prasad, J. Nelson, T. Borus, and W.A. Robinson. 1994. Modification of the effect of Tamoxifen, cis-platin, DTIC and interferon-alpha 2b on human melanoma cells in culture by a mixture of vitamins. *Nutr. Cancer* 22:233-245.

Radin. N.S. 1994. Rationales for cancer chemotherapy with PDMP, a specific inhibitor of lucosylceramide synthase. *Mol. Chem. Neuropathol.* 21:111-127.

Rafferty, J.A., I. Hickson, N. Chinnasamy, L.S. Lashford, G.P. Margison, T.M. Dexter, and L.J. Fairbairn. 1996. Chemoprotection of normal tissues by transfer of drug resistance genes. *Cancer Metastasis Rev.* 15:365-383.

Redman, B.G., Y. Abubakr, T. Chou, P. Esper, and L.E. Flaherty. 1994. Phase II trial of recombinant interleukin-1 beta in patients with metastatic renal cell carcinoma. *J. Immunother. Emphasis Tumor Immunol.* 16:211-215.

Renner, C. and M. Pfreundschuh. 1995. Tumor therapy by immune recruitment with bispecific antibodies. *Immunol. Rev.* 145:179-209.

Research Triangle Institute. 1998. Fact Sheet: RTI's discovery of camptothecin. Research Triangle Institute [Online]. Available: http://www.rti.org/patents/camptothecin.html [May 1998].

Rickinson, A.B. 1995. Immune intervention against virus-associated human cancers. *Ann. Oncol.* **6 Suppl 1**:69-71.

Rischer, C.A. and T.A. Easton. 1995. Cancer. In Focus on Human Biology, 511-522. HarperCollins, New York.

Robins, H.I., D. Rushing, M. Kutz, K.D. Tutsch, C.L. Tiggelaar, D. Paul, D. Spriggs, C. Kraemer, W. Gillis, C. Feierabend, R.Z. Arzoomanian, W. Longo, D. Alberti, F. D'Oleire, R.P. Qu, G. Wilding, and J.A. Stewart. 1997. Phase I clinical trial of melphalan and 41.8 degrees C whole-body hyperthermia in cancer patients. *J. Clin. Oncol.* **15**:158-164.

Roitt, I., J. Brostoff, and D. Male. 1996. Immunology, 4th Ed. Mosby, London.

Rosenthal, D.I. and D.P. Carbone. 1995. Taxol plus radiation for head and neck cancer. *J. Infus. Chemother.* **5**:46-54.

Rougier, P., R. Bugat, J.Y. Douillard, S. Culine, E. Suc, P. Brunet, Y. Becouarn, M. Ychou, M. Marty, J.M. Extra, J. Bonneterre, A. Adenis, J.F. Seitz, G. Ganem, M. Namer, T. Conroy, S. Negrier, Y. Merrouche, F. Burki, M. Mousseau, P. Heirat, and M. Mahjoubi. 1997. Phase II study of irinotecan in the treatment of advanced colorectal cancer in chemotherapy-naive patients and patients pretreated with fluorouracil-based chemotherapy. *J. Clin. Oncol.* **15**:251-260.

Roush, W. 1997a. Antisense aims for a renaissance. *Science* **276**:1192-1193.

Roush, W.1997b. On the biotech pharm, a race to harvest new cancer cures. *Science* **278**:1039-1040.

Saijyo, S., T. Kudo, Y. Katayose, H. Saeki, N. Chiba, M. Suzuki, T. Tominaga, and S. Matsumo. 1996. A new *in vitro* model of specific targeting therapy of cancer: retargeting of PWN-LAK cells with bispecific antibodies greatly enhances cytotoxicity to hepatocellular carcinoma. *Tohoku J. Exp. Med.* **178**:113-127.

Salmon, S.E. and A.C. Sartorelli. 1987. Cancer chemotherapy. In Basic and clinical pharmacology, B.G. Katzung, Ed. 665-701. Appleton and Lange, East Norwalk, Connecticut

Sankaranarayanan, R. and B. Mathew. 1996. Retinoids as cancer-preventive agents. *IARC Sci. Publ.* **(139)**:47-59.

Sankhla, S.K., J.S. Nadkarni, and S.N. Bhagwati. 1996. Adoptive immotherapy using lymphokine-activated killer (LAK) cells and interleukin-2 for recurrent malignant primary brain tumors. *J. Neurooncol.* **27**:133-140.

Santamaria, L., A. Bianchi-Santamaria, and M. Dell'Orti. 1996. Carotenoids in cancer, mastalgia and AIDS:prevention and treatment -- an overview. *J. Environ. Pathol. Toxicol. Oncol.* **15**:89-95.

Sato, T. 1996. Active specific immunotherapy with hapten-modified autologous melanoma cell vaccine. *Cancer Immunol. Immunother.* **43**:174-179.

Schaake-Koning, C., W. van den Bogaert, O. Dalesio, J. Festen, J. Hoogenhout, P. van Houtte, A. Kirkpatrick, M. Koolen, B. Maat, A. Nijs et. al. 1994. Radiosensitization by cytotoxic drugs. The EORTC experience by the Radiotherapy and Lung Cancer Cooperative Groups. *Lung Cancer* **10 Suppl 1**:S263-270.

Schmidt, W., G. Maass, M. Buschle, T. Schweighoffer, M. Berger, E. Herbst, F. Schilcher, and M.L. Birnstiel. 1997. Generation of effective cancer vaccines genetically engineered to secrete cytokines using adenovirus-enhanced transfer infection. *Gene* **190**:211-216.

Schmidt, W., P. Steinlein, M. Buschle, T. Schweighoffer, E. Herbst, K. Mechtler, H. Kirlappos, and M.L. Birnstiel. 1996. Transloading of tumor cells with foreign major histocompatibility complex class I peptide ligand: A novel general strategy for the generation of potent cancer vaccines. *Proc. Natl. Acad. Sci. USA* **93**:9759-9763.

Schneider-Gadicke, E. and G. Riethmuller. 1995. Prevention of manifest metastasis with monoclonal antibodies: a novel approach to immunotherapy of solid tumors. *Eur. J. Cancer* **31A**:1326-1330.

Schuler, M., C. Peschel, F. Schneller, J. Fichtner, L. Flarber, C. Huber, and W.E. Aulitzky. 1996. Immunomodulatory and hematopoietic effects of recombinant human interleukin-6 in patients with advanced renal cell cancer. *J. Interferon Cytokine Res.* **16**:903-910.

Seidman, A.D., C.A. Hudis, G. Rapis, J. Baselga, D. Fennelly, and L. Norton. 1997. Paclitaxel for breast cancer: the Memorial Sloan-Kettering Cancer Center experience. *Oncology (Huntingt)* **11(3 Suppl 2)**: 20-28.

Shchepotin, I.B., D.A. McRae, M. Shabahang, R.R. Buras, and S.R. Evans. 1997. Hyperthermia and verapamil inhibit the growth of human colon cancer xenografts *in vivo* through apoptosis. *Anticancer Res.* 17:2213-2216.

Sidransky, D. 1997. Nucleic-acid based methods for the detection of cancer. *Science* 278:1054-1058.

Sledge, G.W. Jr., M. Qulali, R. Goulet, E.A. Bone, and R. Fife. 1995. Effect of matrix metalloproteinase inhibitor Batimastat on breast cancer regrowth and metastasis in athymic mice. *J. Natl. Cancer Inst.* 87:1546-1550.

Sokoloff, M.H., C.L. Tso, R. Kaboo, S. Taneja, S. Pang, J.B. deKernion, and A.S. Belldegrun. 1996. *In vitro* modulation of tumor progression-associated properties of hormone refractory prostate cell lines by cytokines. *Cancer* 77:1862-1872.

Sone, S. and T. Ogura. 1994. Local interleukin-2 therapy for cancer and its effector induction mechanisms. *Oncology* 51:170-176.

Sredni, B., T. Tichler, A. Shani, R. Catane, B. Kaufman, G. Strassmann, M. Albeck, and Y. Kalechman. 1996. Predominance of TH1 response in tumor-bearing mice and cancer patients treated with AS101. *J. Natl. Cancer Inst.* 88:1276-1284.

Starr, C. And B. McMillan. 1997. Human biology, 2nd Ed. Wadsworth Publishing Co., Belmont, CA.

Stewart, D. 1996. Autologous stem cell transplants. Taking breast and ovarian cancer chemotherapy to new heights. *Medscape Women's Health* 1(7).

Stierle, A., G. Strobel and D. Stierle. 1993. Taxol and taxane production by Taxomyces andreanae, an endophytic fungus of Pacific yew. *Science* 260:214-216.

Sussman, J.J., S. Shu, V.K. Sondak, and A.E. Chang. 1994. Activation of T lymphocytes for the adoptive immunotherapy of cancer. *Ann. Surg. Oncol.* 1:296-306.

Sutedja, T.G. and P.E. Postmus. 1996. Photodynamic therapy in lung cancer. A review. *J Photochem. Photobiol. B* 36:199-204.

Suzuki, K., T. Nakamura, H. Matsuura, K. Kifune and R. Tsurutani. 1995. A new drug delivery system for local cancer chemotherapy using Cisplatin and chitin. *Anticancer Res.* 15:423-426.

Sweetenham, J.W. 1995. The importance of dose and schedule in cancer chemotherapy: haematological cancer. *Anticancer Drugs* **6 Suppl 5**:7-15.

Sweetman, S.F., J.J. Strain, and V.J. McKelvey-Martin. 1997. Effect of antioxidant vitamin supplementation on DNA damage and repair in human lymphoblastoid cells. *Nutr. Cancer* **27**:122-130.

Takahashi, T., N. Mitsuhashi, N. Sakurai, and N. Niibe. 1995. Modifications of tumor-associated antigen expression on human lung cancer cells by hyperthermia and cytokine. *Anticancer Res.* **15**:2601-2606.

Takemura, Y. and A.L. Jackman. 1997. Folate-based thymidylate synthase inhibitors in cancer chemotherapy. *Anticancer Drugs* **8**:3-16.

Takimoto, C.H. and C.J. Allegra. 1995. New antifolates in clinical development. *Oncology (Huntingt)* **9**:649-656.

Tant, C. 1998. Awesome oceans - advances in marine biotechnology. Biotech. Publishing, Angleton, TX. In press.

Teicher, B.A. 1994. Combination of perfluorochemical emulsions and carbogen breathing with cancer chemotherapy. *Artif. Cells Blood Substit. Immobil. Biotechnol.* **22**:1109-1120.

ten Bokkel Huinink, W.W., C.H. Veenhof, M. Huizing, S. Rodenhuis, R. Dubbelman, O. Dalesio, J.H. Beijnen, L. Depauw, and B. Winograd. 1994. Carboplatin and Paclitaxel (Taxol) in patients with advanced ovarian cancer, a dose finding study (Metting abstract). *Ann. Oncol.* **5 (Suppl 8)**:99.

Tepler, I., G. Schwartz, K. Parker, J. Charette, M.E. Kadin, T.G. Woodworth, and L.E. Schnipper. 1994. Phase I trial of an interleukin-2 fusion toxin (DAB486IL-2) in hematologic malignancies: complete response in a patient with Hodgkin's disease refractory to chemotherapy. *Cancer* **73**:1276-1285.

Tetef, M., K. Margolin, C. Ahn, S. Akman, W. Chow, L. Leong, R.J. Morgan Jr., J. Raschko, G. Somlo, and J.H. Doroshow. 1995. Mitomycin C and Menadione for the treatment of lung cancer: a phase II trial. *Invest. New Drugs* **13**:157-162.

Thurnher, M., R. Ramoner, G. Gastl, C. Radmayr, G. Block, M. Herold, H. Klocker, and G. Bartsch. 1997. Bacillus Calmette-Guerinmycobacteria stimulate human blood dendritic cells. *Int. J. Cancer* **70**:128-134.

Tobias, J.S. 1996. The role of radiotherapy in the management of cancer-- an overview. *Ann. Acad. Med. Singapore* **25**:371-379.

Tong, M.C., C.A. van Hasselt, and J.K. Woo. 1996. Preliminary results of photodynamic therapy for recurrent nasopharyngeal carcinoma. *Eur. Arch. Otorhinolaryngol.* **253**:189-192.

Tuting, T., W.J. Storkus, and M.T. Lotze. 1997. Gene-based strategies for the immunotherapy of cancer. *J. Mol. Med.* **75**:478-491.

Uckun, F.M. and G.H. Reaman. 1995. Immunotoxins for the treatment of leukemia and lymphoma. *Leuk. Lymphoma* **18**:195-201.

Unger, C. 1996. Current concepts of treatment in medical oncology: new anticancer drugs. *J. Cancer Res. Clin. Oncol.* **122**:189-198.

van Hillegersberg, R., W.J. Kort, and J.H. Wilson. 1994. Current status of photodynamic therapy in oncology. *Drugs* **48**:510-527.

van Warmerdam, L.J. 1997. Tailor-made chemotherapy for cancer patients. *Neth. J. Med.* **51**:30-35.

VanderWerf, Q.M., R.E. Saxton, A. Chang, D, Horton, M.B. Paiva, J. Anderson, C. Foote, J. Soudant, A. Mathey, and D.J. Castro. 1996. Hypericin: a new laser phototargeting agent fro human cancer cells. *Laryngoscope* **106**:479-483.

Vaughan, W. 1997. Chemotherapy and autologous marrow support for breast cancer . *J.M.C.C.* **4**:14-18 [Online]. Available: http://www.medscape.com/Moffitt/CancerControl/public/archive/1997/0403sup.toc.html [Dec 1997].

Vernon, C.C., J.W. Hand, S.B. Field, D. Machin, J.B. Whaley, J. van der Zee Jr., W.L. Putten, G.C. van Rhoon, J.D. van Dijk, D. Gonzalez Gonzalez, F.F. Liu, P. Goodman, and M. Sherar. 1996. Radiotherapy with or without hyperthermia in the treatment of superficial localized breast cancer: results from five randomized controlled trials. International Collaborative Hyperthermia Group. *Int. J. Radiat. Oncol. Biol. Phys.* **35**:731-744.

Vetrovsky, D.T., L. Gerdom, and G.L. White. 1997. Prostate cancer -- pathology, diagnosis and management. *Clin. Rev.* 7:79-81.

Viloria Petit, A.M., J. Rak, M.-C. Hung, P. Rockwell, N. Goldstein, B. Fendley, and R.S. Kerbel. 1997. Neutralizing antibodies against epidermal growth factor and ErbB-2/neu receptor tyrosine kinases down-regulate vascular endothelial growth factor production by tumor cells *in vitro* and *in vivo. Am. J. Pathol.* 151:1523-1530.

Vink-van Wijngaarden, T., H.A. Pols, C.J. Buurman, G.J. van den Bemd, L.C. Dorssers, J.C. Birkenhlager, and J.P. van Leeuwen. 1994. Inhibition of breast cancer growth by combined treatment with vitamin D3 analogues and Tamoxifen. *Cancer Res.* 54:5711-5717.

Vogel, C.L. 1996. Hormonal approaches to breast cancer treatment and prevention: an overview. *Semin. Oncol.* 23 (4 Suppl 9):2-6.

Voth, E.A. and R.H. Schwartz. 1997. Medicinal applications of delta-9-tetrahydrocannabinol and marijuana. *Ann. Intern. Med.* 126:791-798.

Watson, A. 1997. Photochemotherapy for mycosis fungoides. *Australas. J. Dermatol.* 38:9-11.

Wentworth, P., A. Datta, D. Blakey, T. Boyle, L.J. Partridge, and G.M. Blackburn. 1996. Toward antibody-directed "abzyme" prodrug therapy, ADAPT: carbamate prodrug activation by a catalytic antibody and its in vitro application to human tumor cell killing. *Proc. Natl. Acad. Sci. USA* 93:799-803.

Wersall, P. and H. Mellstedt. 1995. Increased LAK and T cell activation in responding renal cell carcinoma patients after low dose cyclophosphamide, IL-2 and alpha-IFN. *Med. Oncol.* 12:69-77.

Wilking, N., E. Isaksson, and E. von Schoultz. 1997. Tamoxifen and secondary tumours. An update. *Drug Saf.* 16: 104-117.

Williams, N. 1996. Immune boost to the war on cancer. *Science* 272:28-30.

Wills, K.N., D.C. Maneval, P. Menzel, M.P. Harris, S. Sutjipto, M.T. Vaillancourt, W.M. Huang, D.E. Johnson, S.C. Anderson, S.F. Fen et. al. 1994. Development and characterization of recombinant adenoviruses encoding human p53 for gene therapy of cancer. *Hum. Gene Ther.* 5:1079-1088.

Yi, E.S., D. Harclerode, M. Gondo, M. Stephenson, R,W. Brown, M. Younes, and
P.T. Cagle. 1997. High c-erbB-3 protein expression is associated with
shorter survival in advanced non-small cell lung carcinomas. *Mol.
Pathol.* **10**:142-148.

Yuen, A.R., T.J. Panella, T.J. Wieman, C. Julius, M. Panjehpour, S. Taber, V.
Fingar, S.J. Horning, R.A. Miller, S.W. Young, and M.F. Renschler.
1997. Phase I trial of photodynamic therpay with lutetium-Texaphyrin
(LU-TEX) (Abstract). *Proc. Annu. Meet. Am. Soc. Clin. Oncol.*
16:A768.5

Zalutsky, M.R. 1997. Growth factor receptors as molecular targets for cancer
diagnosis and therapy. *Q.J. Nucl. Med.* **41**:71-77.

Zhao, L.R., W.X. Zhao, and M.H. Shao. 1994. [treatment of adv and recurrent
gynecologic cancer by cannula into both internal iliac arteries]. *Chung
Hua Fu Chan Ko Tsa Chih* **29**:607-609.

Zhou, D.C., R. Zittoun, and J.P. Marie. 1995. Homoharringtonine: an effective
new natural product in cancer chemotherapy. *Bull. Cancer (Paris)*
82:987-995.

Zumkeller, W. and P.N. Schofield. 1995. Growth factors, cytokines and soluble
forms of receptor molecules in cancer patients. *Anticancer Res* **15**:343-
348.

Additional references

Ganong, W.F. 1995. Review of medical physiology. Appleton and Lange, East
Norwalk, Connecticut.

Lewin, B.1990. Genes IV. Cell Press, Cambridge, MA and Oxford University
Press, New York.

Glossary

active gene - a gene which is "turned on" and is making messenger RNA for translation into protein

adjuvant - a chemical added to a vaccine which improves the immune response to the vaccine

aggressive - likely to spread and grow rapidly

amino acid - chemical component of a protein

androgens - male reproductive hormones, including testosterone and dihydrotestosterone

angiogenesis - the formation of new blood vessels

antibody - Y shaped protein made by the immune system which can attach to antigens

anti-oxidant - chemical which can neutralize free radicals

antigen - chemical recognized by the immune system, in particular by lymphocytes or antibodies

antigen presenting cell - a cell that shows antigens to a helper T cell and (usually) turns it on

apoptosis - suicide of a cell in response to certain stimuli

B cell - white blood cell (immune cell) which makes antibodies

base - one of the four chemical components of DNA or RNA - adenine, guanine, cytosine, or thymine

benign tumor - tumor which is not expected to metastasize or be dangerous to life

bone marrow - tissue inside the bones, where all cells of the blood are made

carcinogen - chemical which promotes the development of cancer

cell cycle - a series of "life stages" for a cell, from G1 (resting) through cell division

cell cycle genes - genes which control a cell's progress through the cell cycle

cell division - splitting each cell into two new cells

chemoprevention - the prevention of cancer with drugs

chromosome - a long strand of DNA which carries the genes

circadian - in a 24-hour cycle

colon - the large intestine, a part of the digestive tract

complete regression - complete disappearance of a tumor, whether temporary or permanent

cyclins - proteins which control the progress of a cell through the cell cycle

cytoplasm - the contents of a cell which are contained within the cell membrane but outside the nucleus

cytotoxic drug - drug which can kill a cell

cytotoxic T cell - type of lymphocyte which specializes in killing abnormal body cells, especially virus infected cells and cancer cells

cytokine - protein made by the immune system which carries instructions to other cells

daughter cells - the new cells produced after a cell divides

detoxify - render harmless

differentiation - the process by which a cell "grows up" and becomes a mature cell

endothelial cells - cells found lining the inside of a blood vessel, which migrate into a tumor to form a new blood vessel

enzymes - specialized proteins which speed chemical reactions and make reactions possible which would not otherwise occur

epithelial tissue - layers of cells which usually line body surfaces and form glands

extracellular matrix - proteins and other substances which surround cells

fragile site - site in the chromosome which is more likely to break than most areas

free radicals - chemicals with an extra electron, which have a tendency to react with other molecules in the cell and destroy them

growth factor - a molecule which stimulates cells to divide

helper T cell - type of lymphocyte which makes cytokines and specializes in helping other cells of the immune system

hormone - chemical messenger in the body, sent to cells to control their functions

hypoxic - low in oxygen

ion - an atom with either a positive or negative charge

immunotoxin - an antibody molecule which carries a drug, toxin, or radioactive molecule

LAK cell - lymphocyte from the blood which has been stimulated with cytokines; contains Natural Killer cells and other types of cells

leukemia - a cancer of the red or white blood cells

lymph nodes - collections of lymphocytes along lymphatic vessels, where most immune reactions occur

lymphatic vessels - small tubes which resemble blood vessels, but carry a fluid called lymph from the tissues to the blood

lymphocyte - a type of immune (white blood) cell

macrophage - a white blood cell (immune cell) which destroys bacteria and abnormal body cells, and presents antigens

malignant tumor - a cancer

median - a statistical measurement often used in cancer treatment. To get the median, list the values from lowest to highest, and select the value in the middle

messenger RNA - a string of bases which carries the instructions to make a protein (from the gene to the protein manufacturing apparatus in the cytoplasm)

gene - a piece of DNA which carries the information to make a protein

metastasis - spread of cancer cells from the original tumor to more distant parts of the body

MHC I molecule - a molecule (found on all cells of the body) which displays antigens for cytotoxic T cells

MHC II molecule - a molecule (found only on antigen presenting cells) which displays antigens for helper T cells

microtubules - small tubes (made up of tubulins) inside the cell which transport substances, help to maintain the cell's shape, and move the chromosomes to the new cells during cell division

mitosis - cell division resulting in two new cells with the same genes as the original cell

mutagens - substances which are able to cause mutations in DNA

mutation - a change in the order of bases in DNA or a break in a chromosome

Natural Killer cell - a type of lymphocyte which can kill abnormal cells such as virus-infected cells and cancer cells.

neutrophil - a type of white blood cell which mainly kills bacteria

nucleus - the membrane-enclosed portion of a cell where the genes are found

nutrient - something that nourishes; the sugars and other molecules which provide nutrition for cells and for the body in general

oncogene - a gene which promotes cancer

ovary - the organ in a woman which makes eggs, and the hormones estrogen and progesterone

p53 - a tumor suppressor protein (made from the p53 gene) which stops the cell cycle and may stimulate apoptosis in the cell

partial regression - a partial shrinkage of a tumor

peptide - small piece of a protein

photosensitizer - drug which kills cells by generating free radicals when it is exposed to light

platelet - fragment of a cell which initiates blood clotting

premalignant site - an area where cells are abnormal but not yet cancerous

radiosensitizer - chemical which makes a cell more sensitive to radiation

prodrug - drug which is non-toxic to cells, but which can be converted into a toxic drug by certain enzymes

receptor - molecule which serves as an attachment site for another molecule. Usually, it sends a message to the cell when its partner attaches

red blood cell - the cell which carries oxygen in the blood

remission - a period of time during which the symptoms of cancer diminish or disappear

stem cells - cells in the bone marrow which make blood cells

telomerases - the enzymes which elongate the ends of the chromosomes

telomeres - the ends of the chromosomes

testes - the organ in a man which makes sperm and testosterone

tissue - organized group of cells and proteins

toxic - harmful to the body or to a cell

toxin - poison

tumor infiltrating lymphocytes (TILs) - lymphocytes found in and around the tumor, which can be taken out of the body, stimulated, and returned to the patient to fight the cancer

tumor suppressor genes - genes which suppress cancers until they are mutated

white blood cell - cell which fights infections and abnormal cells such as cancer; immune cell

Trade Names

Many of the drugs used in cancer treatment and research have become known by tradenames used by the drug producer. Since these are the names most likely to be encountered by both the lay reader and physician, we have used them instead of the technical chemical name. They are used in this manner fir the benefit of their owner or developer and should not be used as common nouns. Such names are listed below along with some generic names. In some cases the original literature cited did not distinguish trade and generic names and did not provide manufacturer information.

Adriamycin	Lupron
Alkeran	Methotrexate
Angiostatin	Mutamycin
Batimastat	Mythramycin
Buspar	Nilutamide
Bryostatin 1	Oncovin
Carboplatin	Paclitaxel
Cerubidine	Photofrin
Cisplatin	Plachitin
Cytasar	Platinol
Cytotoxin	Purinethol
Docetaxel	Raloxifene
Doxorubicin	Roidex
Endostatin	Sulindac
Eniposide	Tamoxifen
Ethiofos	Taxol
Etoposide	Texaphyrin
Fentretinate	Thalidomide
Finasteride	Thapsigargin
Fludarabine	Tomudex
Flutamide	Topotecan (Hycamtin)
Ganciclovir	Trofosfamide
Hypericin	Velban
Leukeran	Vincristine
Levamisole	Zoladex
Lu-Tex	

Index

A

5-fluorouracil 58, 76, 82, 95, 106, 202

ADAPT 18, 104, 276

adjuvant 45, 220, 225, 254, 259, 263, 278

alkylating agents 72, 170

androgens 125, 127-131, 171, 179, 244, 278

anemia 8, 85

anthracyclines 73, 74, 90

antibodies 53, 97-102, 104, 114, 120-123, 149, 183, 190, 193, 194, 196, 199, 200, 205, 207, 211-215, 255, 257-259, 261, 270-272, 276, 278

antibody 71, 97-102, 104, 120, 190, 191, 199, 200, 205, 212-214, 253, 262, 270, 276, 278, 280

antigen presenting cell 187, 210, 278

antigens 97, 182-187, 189, 190, 193, 194, 200, 209-212, 214, 215, 218-220, 222, 224-226, 249, 260, 263, 278, 280, 281

antioxidants 244, 246, 260

antisense molecules 236-239

APC 37, 40, 43, 67, 248, 249

apoptosis 38, 50, 114, 123, 168, 171-179, 195, 235, 238, 248, 250, 256, 257, 260-262, 267, 273, 278, 281

aromatase inhibitors 134, 255

asparaginase 84

B

B cell .... 101, 190, 263, 278 bases 10, 12, 13, 15, 23, 58, 72-74, 76, 236, 237, 257, 281

Batimastat 143, 258, 273

BCG 201, 257

Bcl-2 . . . . 177, 179, 238

BEHAB 142

benign tumors 2

beta carotene 135, 245-247

bispecific 213-215, 253, 270, 271

blood cells 2, 6, 10, 33, 53, 85-88, 97, 109, 110, 145, 151, 165, 181, 203, 280, 282

blood clots 128, 154, 243

blood vessels 6, 43, 55, 93, 94, 96, 100, 101, 122, 140, 141, 147-156, 158, 168, 202, 253, 278, 280

bone marrow 7, 53, 85-88, 92, 99, 105, 109, 110, 113, 114, 136, 165, 181-184, 231, 256, 267, 278, 282

brachytherapy 52

BRCA1 and BRCA2 39

breast cancer 2, 20, 29, 37, 39, 62, 67, 77, 79, 80, 100, 110-112, 114, 115, 120, 123-125, 130-134, 139, 141, 150, 155, 169, 170, 243, 244, 248, 252, 254, 255, 257, 258, 261-268, 270, 272, 273, 275, 276

Bryostatin-1 143

C

cadherin 141

camptothecin 77, 271

carbogen 56, 262, 268, 274

Carboplatin 72, 82, 95, 274

carcinogens 18-20, 23, 241, 252

carotenoids 135, 137, 245, 272

castration 127-129

cell cycle 27-30, 32, 35, 37-39, 42, 58, 174, 176, 227, 278, 279, 281

cell-mediated immunity 190, 191, 205, 213

cervical cancer 20, 42, 58, 241, 249

chemoprevention 242, 249, 254, 262, 268, 279

chemotherapy 45, 62, 67, 71-73, 79, 85, 87-89, 92, 95, 96, 106, 109-115, 123, 127, 132, 152-155, 163, 165, 169-171, 177-179, 201, 202, 204, 208, 213, 214, 226, 250, 253-256, 258-263, 265, 266, 268-271, 273-275, 277

chromosomes 9, 10, 12, 15, 18, 21, 23, 39-41, 74, 78, 230, 281, 282

circadian rhythms 105-107, 259

Cisplatin 72, 82, 86, 96, 106, 123, 144, 260, 273

clinical trials 45, 62, 68-70, 76-79, 81, 92, 96, 106, 107, 111, 122, 129, 133, 136,137, 149-151, 160, 163, 169, 177, 180, 203, 206, 208, 213, 223, 229, 231, 238, 245, 247-249, 259, 266, 267

colon cancer 2, 37, 40, 67, 76, 77, 104, 107, 124, 169, 213, 222, 225, 233, 248, 273

co-stimulation 187, 210, 256

cyclin 28, 29, 32, 42, 176

cyclin-dependent kinases 28, 29, 32, 42

cyclophosphamide 72, 82, 86-88, 276

cytokines 88, 183, 186-188, 190, 193, 194, 200-209, 220, 236, 254, 263, 267, 272, 273, 277, 280

cytotoxic T cell 188, 190, 279

D

dendritic cell 187

dihydrotestosterone 125, 127, 128, 130, 244, 278

disintegrins 145

DNA 9-11, 13, 15, 18-20, 23, 24, 27, 29, 30, 32, 37-40, 42, 43, 50, 58, 71-77, 84, 88, 91, 92, 109, 114, 123, 158, 163, 169, 172, 174, 176, 178, 179, 225, 236, 238, 239, 246, 264, 274, 278, 279, 281

Docetaxel 78, 79, 81, 82, 253, 264

Doxorubicin 73, 80, 86, 90, 103, 104, 106, 155, 178, 267

drug resistance 85, 89-93, 155, 231, 257, 259, 270

E

eleutherobin 83

epidermal growth factor 30, 32, 33, 117, 119, 120, 254, 276

epothilones 83, 84, 268

Erythropoietin 88

estrogen 10, 114, 128, 131-134, 243, 256, 263, 281

external 51, 163, 173, 174

F

Fas 172, 173, 175, 178, 179, 195, 196, 262

fibroblasts 55, 156

Finasteride 130, 244

Flutamide 129, 130, 244

free radicals 50, 55-57, 60, 135, 158, 244, 246, 278, 280, 282

FSH 125, 126, 130

G

gamma rays 50, 51

gene delivery viruses 229

gene marker studies 232, 239

gene therapy 45, 58, 92, 114, 122, 227-232, 234-236, 239, 250, 252, 261, 262, 269, 276

GM-CSF 88, 223

GnRH 125, 126, 128-131

goserelin 128, 129, 244, 255

growth factors 4, 17, 30, 31, 43, 117-120, 144, 148-150, 156, 177, 178, 213, 277

G-CSF 88

H

hapten-modified 222, 254, 272

helper T cell 183, 185, 187, 188, 210, 278, 280

HER-2 .... 30, 33, 100, 119, 121-123, 214, 225, 226, 258, 262

high dose 109-115, 165

HIMAC 52

homoharringtonine 84, 277

hormones 8, 30, 71, 125-127, 129, 130, 201, 242, 278, 281

humanized 101, 102

hydroxyurea 58, 76

hyperbaric 56

hyperthermia 93, 165, 167-171, 250, 259, 260, 267, 270, 271, 273-275

I

ifosfamide 72

immortality genes 42

immunotoxins 53, 98-100, 104, 263, 275

in cancer prevention 23, 137, 241, 244, 246

in phototherapy 158, 161, 162

inhibitors 32, 76, 77, 134, 143, 148, 150-153, 177, 242, 243, 248, 255, 260, 268, 274

insulin-like growth factor 1 124

interferon 115, 163, 202-204, 206, 223, 252, 261, 264, 270, 272

interleukin-2 .... 188, 203, 258, 261, 270, 272-274

interleukin-6 .... 257, 258, 272

internal 25, 26, 31-33, 42, 50-53, 96, 105, 167, 169, 174, 277

irinotecan 77, 271

K

kidney cancer 107, 204

L

lasers 160, 167, 267

leukemia 2, 18, 20, 21, 84, 99, 107, 136, 179, 203, 206, 233, 264, 275, 280

leuprolide 128

LH .... 125, 126, 128-131 liposomes 229, 230, 234, 235

lung cancer 1, 20, 88, 241, 245-247, 272-274

LY353381 . . . . 133, 243

lymph nodes 112, 140, 184, 187, 222, 280

lymphatic vessels 6, 140, 184, 280

M

macrophage 159, 181, 263, 280

MAGE proteins 219

mdr-1 gene 92

medical 52, 80, 127-129, 148, 275, 277

melanoma 81, 89, 137, 170, 199, 222, 223, 225, 235, 252, 254,
258, 260, 262, 266, 269, 270, 272

melatonin 88, 265

metalloproteinases 143

metastasis 6, 43, 47, 48, 50, 57, 110, 112, 128, 139-141, 143-145,
150, 201, 213, 222, 223, 235, 254, 257, 258, 270, 272, 273, 281

MHC I molecules 188, 189, 194, 222

MHC II molecules 186

microtubules 77-80, 83, 84, 89, 178, 281

monoclonal 102, 114, 212-214, 259, 261, 272

MORF4 42

mutations 1, 3-5, 10, 12, 17-20, 23-25, 27, 30, 31, 35, 37-40, 42,
43, 47, 48, 50, 72, 174, 176, 206, 227, 235, 281

N

naked DNA 225

Natural Killer cell 193, 202, 281

necrosis 171-173, 204, 209, 257

neutrophil 88, 281

nm23 . . . . 141, 269

non-specific immunostimulators 201, 207

O

oncogenes 17, 21, 22, 24-26, 29-33, 35, 42-44, 47, 67, 227,
231, 236, 259

ovarian cancer 79-81, 113, 114, 214, 233, 238, 256, 258, 262, 264,
267, 273, 274

oxygen 6, 10, 53, 55-57, 60, 109, 147, 153, 154, 158, 159,
163, 168, 170,174, 178, 280, 282

P

p53 . . . . 29, 37, 38, 40, 42, 43, 47, 48, 50, 114, 123, 174-180,
227, 235, 253, 257, 260, 265, 276, 281

Paclitaxel 62, 78-84, 86, 92, 106, 252, 253, 255, 261, 262,
267, 268, 272, 274

Pgp proteins 91

phase I trials 69, 143

phase II trials 69, 77

phase III trials 69

phototherapy 57, 114, 157-165, 250, 264

Plachitin 96

platelets 85, 87, 109, 145

porphycenes 160-162

porphyrins 57, 160, 161, 259

preclinical trials 93, 100, 220, 231, 235, 238

premalignant lesions 242, 247

prodrugs 103, 104

prostate cancer 62, 118, 124, 125, 127, 129, 130, 137, 179, 244, 252, 254-256, 259, 276

protein and peptide 224, 225

protein synthesis 13, 84

R

radiation 18-20, 23, 39, 43, 45, 49-60, 62, 123, 127, 129, 1 52, 161,163, 165, 169, 171, 177, 178, 201, 241, 250, 255, 259, 269, 271, 282

radiosensitizers 55, 57-59

Raloxifene 133, 243

ras 31-33, 43, 47, 48, 238, 269

red 2, 10, 53, 85, 87, 88, 109, 168, 232, 248, 280, 282

remissions 70, 115, 132, 203, 213, 224

repair 20, 23, 24, 38, 39, 42, 43, 58, 72, 74, 84, 91, 92, 169, 176, 178, 274

resistance 55, 56, 85, 89-93, 151, 155, 231, 257, 259, 260, 266, 268-270

retinoblastoma 35, 37, 38, 67, 227

retinoids 135-137, 144, 171, 178, 247, 248, 257, 272

ribozymes 236, 238, 239

S

sensitization 58

side effects 52-55, 57, 65, 68, 69, 71, 76, 78, 82, 85-88, 92, 95, 96, 98, 101, 103, 106-109, 113, 128, 129, 134, 137, 143, 158-163, 169, 180, 202, 203, 205, 207, 209, 213, 226, 231, 235, 238, 243, 244, 248, 249

single chain toxins 100

squamous cell carcinoma 204, 248

stem cells 85, 86, 92, 109, 110, 113-115, 165, 282

suicide genes 232, 236, 239

suppression of 179

suramin 118, 150

T

Tamoxifen 62, 131-134, 243, 248, 263-265, 270, 276

telomerases 40-42, 282

testosterone 125-131, 244, 278, 282

Texaphyrins 56, 57, 161

Thalidomide 151, 152

to lymph nodes 140

topoisomerase inhibitors 76, 77

Topotecan 77, 95

TRAIL 173-175, 179, 261

transfusions 87, 88

Trofosfamide . . . . 72, 255 tumor infiltrating lymphocytes (TILs) 282

tumor suppressor genes 24, 25, 30, 35, 37-40, 42-44, 47, 227, 231, 235, 236, 239, 282

U

urokinase 144

V

vaccines 122, 123, 217-226, 228, 231, 239, 249, 266, 272

vinblastine 78

vinca alkaloids 78, 79, 86, 89, 90

Vincristine 78, 106

viruses 18, 20, 21, 23, 25, 87, 122, 171, 182, 190, 199, 217, 222, 229, 230, 234, 235, 249

virus-modified 222

vitamins 45, 135, 137, 244, 246, 247, 268, 270

W

white 2, 85, 87, 88, 97, 109, 136, 163, 165, 181, 203, 257, 259, 264, 276, 278, 280-282